Comments on *Irritable Bowel Syndrome: Answers at your fingertips* from readers:

'Very readable and comprehensive . . . also good at allaying reasonable fears that IBS sufferers may have. I would recommend it.'

SARA SELMES
Development Officer, IBS Network

'A very informative book; a resource that can be frequently used to refer to for advice.'

MARY HASLAM SRN
Senior Nurse Manager, Medical Advisory Service

'I have suffered from IBS since I was a teenager. I feel I understand the condition much better after reading this book. And it is really reassuring to discover I am normal!'

MRS R DIXON
Sussex

Irritable Bowel Syndrome

Answers at your fingertips

Dr Udi Shmueli MD FRCP

Consultant Physician and Gastroenterologist,
Northampton General Hospital

CLASS PUBLISHING · LONDON

Printing history
First published 2007, reprinted 2011

The author and publishers welcome feedback from the users of this book. Please contact the publishers.

Class Health, The Exchange, Express Park, Bristol Road, Bridgwater, TA6 4RR, UK
Telephone: 020 7371 2119
Fax: 020 7371 2878 [International +4420]
email: post@class.co.uk
www.class.co.uk

The information presented in this book is accurate and current to the best of the author's knowledge. The author and publisher, however, make no guarantee as to, and assume no responsibility for, the correctness, sufficiency or completeness of such information or recommendation. The reader is advised to consult a doctor regarding all aspects of individual health care.

A CIP catalogue record for this book is available from the British Library

ISBN 13: 9781859593288

Edited by Carrie Walker

Designed and typeset by Martin Bristow

Cartoons by Jane Taylor

Printed and bound in Great Britain by the MPG Books Group

Contents

Dedication
To my father, and his bowel

About the author and contributor

Dr Ehoud Shmueli (usually known as Udi) MD, FRCP, is Consultant Physician and Gastroenterologist at Northampton General Hospital.

Chapter 11, on Psychological Aspects of IBS, has been jointly authored by Udi Shmueli and Avi Shmueli.

Avi Shmueli PhD, Dip Clin Psychol, trained initially as a clinical psychologist and then as a psychoanalyst. He now works in full-time private practice at the Anna Freud Centre and at the Tavistock Centre for Couple Relationships. Avi is an Honorary Senior Lecturer at University College London, and combines individual and couple therapies with additional responsibilities for teaching and research.

Foreword

by **Kathleen McGrath**
*Director of Medical Services and Vice-Chairman,
Medical Advisory Service.*

We live in a society in which almost any subject is now openly discussed. Sexual orientation/health, mental illness and handicap are among those issues covered regularly in the media. Sadly this is not the case when it comes to the taboo of bowel health and function. For some reason, we remain squeamish about communicating our concerns about the signs and symptoms of bowel disorders. Embarrassment and fear often prevent patients from seeking professional help with common bowel problems.

The Medical Advisory Service has, for over 10 years, been meeting the needs of patients with possible irritable bowel syndrome (IBS), encouraging them, through a specialist nurse-run helpline, to seek diagnosis and help. The impact of IBS on people's daily lives is widely reported and documented; sufferers are often dragged down by the effort to self-manage, to find the nearest loo and to cope with cramping stomach pain. Reference books like this are to be welcomed as they provide accessible information and support to patients and their carers. This volume genuinely fills a communication gap that often exists between patients and healthcare professionals – especially in the case of life-long conditions.

A diagnosis of IBS is really only the start of an individual's journey. Ongoing management and information on options in treatment are essential tools in managing symptoms and getting on with leading a more normal and fulfilling life. This positive guide is an ideal first step in achieving better bowel health.

Katheen McGrath

Acknowledgements

I would like to thank my friends and colleagues at Northampton General Hospital for their help, encouragement and support, but particularly for making Northampton a pleasant place to work, leaving me with the enthusiasm to write this book.

I would also like to thank my brother Avi for the chapter on the psychological aspects of IBS.

Thank you to everyone who read and commented on the book, particularly to the people at the IBS Network for their comments and suggestions.

A big thank you to the people at Class Publishing, in particular to Richard Warner for his enthusiasm, advice and patience, Carrie Walker for the excellent editing, and our artist, Jane Taylor, for the wonderful cartoons.

Introduction

To eat is human. To digest divine.
Mark Twain

Most of us eat and drink without worrying about our digestion and defecation. This book is intended for those whose life is affected by the symptoms of irritable bowel syndrome (IBS): bloating, abdominal pain, diarrhoea and constipation. For some people, IBS is a trivial complaint, the equivalent of some people's tension headaches. For others, it comes to dominate their lives.

This suffering may be compounded by the derisory attitude adopted towards IBS by some health professionals and some lay people. Nobody dies of IBS, so it might be seen as a trivial complaint blown out of all proportion by depressed pathetic people. But this isn't so. It's easy to feel isolated with IBS despite the fact that it may afflict up to 20% of the population.

People with IBS should understand that, historically, blaming the victim was a common response to insoluble problems. I believe that the attitude of health professionals, the media and the public in general towards IBS has greatly improved in recent years. In part this reflects the realisation of just how common a condition it is in all societies, but mostly it reflects our greater understanding of IBS as a condition. We are better able to diagnose and treat IBS than ever before. The future holds greater promise.

Today there are many websites that provide useful information for people with health problems. An excellent recent addition is the Self Management Programme for IBS available from the IBS Network (see the Appendix for contact details). People should be encouraged to explore such sites and try for themselves different strategies and treatments. Even if you don't have the confidence to try things recommended by a website, having some understanding and just knowing what the treatment options are will help you get the best from your doctor.

One aim of this book is to take your knowledge of IBS one step further. It answers questions in more detail and depth than is usually available from help leaflets and websites. It does not promote a single solution. Rather, it explains the 'physiology' and 'pharmacology' behind currently available treatments – that is, how they affect the body – encouraging and empowering people to try different strategies to reduce the impact of IBS on their lives.

The book is a series of questions and answers. It can be read from cover to cover, but most people will prefer to dip in and out of the different sections, looking for answers to their own questions. There are, however, three main questions that people ask about IBS:

- What causes IBS?

- Can I be sure that I don't have something else?

- What can I do about IBS?

WHAT CAUSES IBS?

One of the objectives of this book is to describe the science behind IBS.

The cause of IBS isn't known yet. It is defined as a syndrome – a collection of symptoms – rather than a disease. Some people feel that doctors use it as a 'dustbin diagnosis': if they can't find anything wrong, they say a person has IBS – a longer-lasting version of the famous 'virus' that doctors blame undiagnosable complaints on, just to get the patient out of the surgery! There is in fact some truth in this, as IBS is to some extent a 'diagnosis of exclusion'. There is no test for IBS, and it is diagnosed when tests for other conditions are negative. However, the absence of a medical test to diagnose IBS in the clinic *does not mean* that IBS is not a real condition.

In IBS, the function of the bowel is disturbed, causing symptoms, but its structure is normal. We are beginning to understand how this occurs, and one of the objectives of this book is to describe the science behind IBS, and the sophisticated techniques being used to understand symptoms such as bloating and pain. Based on our increasing understanding of the pathways that the gut and the brain use to communicate, new drugs are and will be emerging to target specific groups of people with IBS.

One of the first steps in understanding the cause of a medical problem is to define the *epidemiology* – that means who gets the condition and what other conditions is it associated with. This is discussed in Chapter 2. There are many hypotheses to explain IBS and some of these are discussed in Chapter 3, including the leading medical hypothesis of 'visceral hypersensitivity'. This is the idea that IBS involves disordered signalling between the gut and the brain. Signals from the gut become overamplified so that signals usually meaning normal function, which a person is hardly aware of, show up instead as pain. The disordered signalling leads to disordered function, with diarrhoea, bloating and constipation. How and why this disordered signalling occurs is unknown, but various factors may contribute, including infection, persisting inflammation and psychological stress.

Chapter 6 describes what we know about the mechanism of bloating. This was once thought to be a problem of the large bowel, but it is now recognised as a disorder of the small bowel.

Chapter 7 looks at the causes of constipation and the contribution of dietary fibre. Some people think that 'Thou should eat more fibre' ought to be the eleventh commandment. In fact, only a small proportion of people with IBS will benefit from more dietary fibre.

Chapter 8 looks at some of the many possible causes of diarrhoea. Unfortunately, conditions such as coeliac disease are still being misdiagnosed as IBS.

Chapter 10 looks at food allergy and intolerance as a cause of IBS or a factor contributing to it. Simple changes to the diet occasionally result in profound benefit. At other times, people make a huge effort in a fruitless search for the right diet.

Chapter 11 examines the psychological contribution to IBS. Some people see the gut as a 'metaphor for the mind' – psychological turmoil playing itself out in the coils of the intestine! Certainly, the old dichotomy between mind and body no longer applies and is, for IBS, fairly useless as a concept.

CAN I BE SURE THAT I DON'T HAVE SOMETHING ELSE?

People who have had symptoms for more than 6 months without anything obvious developing, such as weight loss or persistent bleeding, are unlikely to have a serious condition. Most people with IBS have had symptoms for years. Even so, during a bad episode, it is natural to wonder if something else has developed.

There are several approaches to dealing with such worries. You might try to ignore them, at least for a while. This is a very reasonable strategy, especially if you have had IBS for a long time and know that your symptoms will come and go. As soon as you feel better, you'll feel very relieved. Another approach is to think of all the other times you thought you were going to die, and laugh at yourself. I myself had several 'terminal illnesses' at medical school but I'm still here!

Alternatively, you could seek reassurance from a professional. Simple direct reassurance from a trusted professional may be enough for some. However, I believe that many people need to understand something of the knowledge on which such reassurance is based. To help you with this, Chapter 4 describes the pain of IBS, while Chapter 5 describes the symptoms of some other conditions and how to distinguish them from IBS. Whether you find the descriptions of other conditions helpful or whether you talk yourself into having these conditions depends on your personality. In any case, you will be left with a greater understanding of how doctors differentiate between different conditions.

People worry most about pain, but it is actually diarrhoea that is most frequently misdiagnosed. Chapter 8 therefore discusses at length conditions that cause diarrhoea and may be mistaken for IBS.

WHAT CAN I DO ABOUT IBS?

There are many relatively simple treatments to try.

People use different strategies to deal with ongoing IBS symptoms. Many people just accept their symptoms, live with them and ignore them as much as possible so that the symptoms are not in control of their lives. This is probably a very successful strategy as we know that many people in the general population who have IBS never consult a doctor and are happy with simple medications or no treatment at all.

Some people go to the other extreme and embark on a search for a 'magic bullet' to treat them. They go from doctor to doctor, alternative practitioner to alternative practitioner, looking for the right test or the right treatment to sort them out. To a certain extent, this approach may work. The placebo effect – the response to a sham, dummy or pretend treatment – is very powerful in IBS. So if you believe that a treatment will work, there is about a 50% chance that it will. The placebo effect can last for 3 months. Hence every time you see another practitioner, of whatever kind, who 'sells' you his or her favourite treatment, you may get 3 months' relief.

Modern doctors probably don't make sufficient use of the placebo effect. It does after all show something very exciting about the power of positive thought. We are, however, a little obsessed with 'evidence-based medicine'. Rather than simply telling people that the treatment will make them better, we tend to weaken the effect by explaining that it works in a proportion of people, and here are the side effects. People looking for a magic bullet are usually disappointed. The plethora of books, websites, miracle diets and complementary medicines for IBS all highlight the fact that there isn't a cure. But different approaches work well for different people, and the trick is finding what's best for you.

This book employs a 'symptom-orientated' approach to pain, bloating, diarrhoea and constipation. This mean that various approaches to dealing with these symptoms are suggested in different chapters. If one symptom is worse for you, it might therefore be useful to start with that chapter to find some new ideas for dealing with it.

People are often willing to try complementary medicines for IBS but are more reluctant to consider a psychological approach. Both, however, are worth considering. Indeed, cognitive behavioural therapy and hypnosis may be two of the most successful approaches to reducing the effects of IBS on quality of life. These are discussed along with other psychological and complementary approaches in Chapters 11 and 12.

WHAT ABOUT DIET AND IBS?

The role of diet in disease has been food for debate for centuries. 'Let food be thy medicine, thy medicine shall be thy food', said Hippocrates. And 'He that takes medicine and neglects diet, wastes the skill of the physician' is an old Chinese proverb. You might argue that the only part of your digestive tract that you truly control is the first 7 centimetres – control it well and your problems will be solved! But the truth is far more complex.

People looking for a diet to solve the problems of IBS may be disappointed. Dietary measures can help some people some of the time, but there is usually a great deal of trial and error. Variability between individuals and within the same individual over time makes it difficult to give dietary advice. The idea that all people with IBS just need a little more fibre in their diet has been dismissed, and the role of fibre is discussed mainly in the chapter on constipation. That said, a little more fibre or other dietary alterations do work for some people.

Food allergies and intolerance, a source of great controversy, are discussed in Chapter 10, where different types of elimination diets are presented.

HOW ACCURATE IS THIS BOOK?

'Half of what we know is untrue. The problem is – which half?' This saying was quoted in one of my first medical textbooks, and it is as true of this book as of any other. Nevertheless, the book is based on my experience as a gastroenterologist treating people with IBS and other gastroenterological complaints, as well as on the published medical literature. I would welcome any feedback readers wish to provide. Not everyone will agree with the answers that I give, but the book can only be improved if you let me know when you disagree and have found my advice to be unhelpful. I would also like to know if there are important questions that have not been covered. Please write to me c/o Class publishing, Barb House, Barb Mews, London W6 7PA, UK.

FINALLY . . .

The final word comes from Mark Twain – 'Be careful about reading health books. You may die of a misprint'!

1 | How the gut works – the normal effects of food

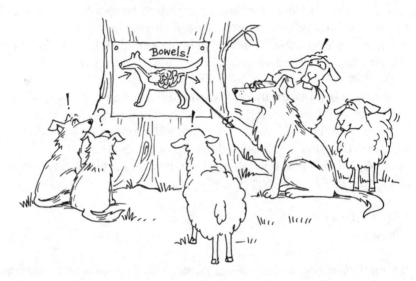

The gastrointestinal tract is made up of the mouth, oesophagus, stomach, small bowel and large bowel. It digests and absorbs the food and holds what's left until we are ready to expel it when we defecate. To understand the 'how and why' of medical treatment and investigation for irritable bowel syndrome (IBS), it's important to have an idea of the basic structure and function of the gastrointestinal tract.

THE MOUTH

My mum used to tell me off for not chewing my food properly. Is chewing important?

Chewing reduces the size of the pieces of food so that they can be swallowed. Eating quickly will probably have little effect on the digestion of most foods as long as you chew well enough, but it will result in more air being swallowed. Even when we just swallow a little saliva, a few millilitres of air will go down too. If we gulp down our food, we will inevitably swallow more air.

We now believe that the bloating experienced in IBS is mostly due to excess air in the small bowel. Most of this air is swallowed. Hence if you suffer from bloating, eating slowly and chewing well may be important.

How much saliva do we make in a day?

About 1.5 litres (3 pints) of saliva are produced each day. The secretion of saliva is stimulated by food – so if no food is eaten, only 500 ml will be produced. Sleep, fatigue, fear and dehydration all reduce the secretion of saliva.

What does saliva do?

Saliva keeps the lining of the mouth moist and lubricates the food. It is alkaline to protect the teeth from acidic food and also contains an antibacterial enzyme. In addition, the digestion of carbohydrates begins in the mouth with the salivary enzyme amylase.

THE OESOPHAGUS

The oesophagus is a tube about 25 centimetres (10 inches) long that carries food from the mouth to the stomach (Figure 1.1).

What can go wrong with the oesophagus?

Reflux of acid from the stomach up into the oesophagus seems to be getting more common, producing indigestion symptoms such as heartburn, chest pain, pain in the upper abdomen and difficulty swallowing. In severe cases of reflux, there can be ulceration and

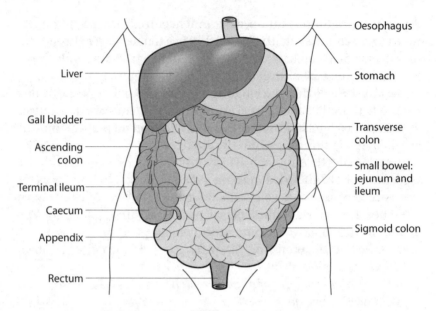

Figure 1.1 The abdominal digestive system.

bleeding. Cancer of the oesophagus is often first noticed because a person has difficulty swallowing (dysphagia). It is associated with smoking, alcohol consumption and acid reflux. Difficulty swallowing is also sometimes due to poor co-ordination of the muscles in the oesophagus.

THE STOMACH

The chest and the abdomen are separated by a dome-shaped sheet of muscle called the diaphragm. This is the chief muscle used in breathing in (inspiration). When it contracts, the contents of the abdomen are compressed down while the chest cavity is enlarged, drawing air into the lungs. Clearly, when the stomach is full, it becomes more difficult for the diaphragm to work, which is why it's easier to exercise on an empty stomach.

The diaphragm has an opening in its centre through which the oesophagus empties into the stomach. The stomach is a J-shaped bag with an average capacity of 1 litre (2 pints; Figure 1.1). It is, however, capable of a lot of expansion (called dilatation), to hold food for the first processes of digestion and then to release it in a controlled fashion to the small bowel. Interestingly, the stomach can distinguish between fluids and solids, so that fluids taken on an empty stomach may pass straight through into the duodenum.

Functionally, the stomach works in two halves. The upper part expands to hold the food coming down from the oesophagus. It therefore acts as a reservoir of food for the lower part of the stomach. The lower part is controlled by a pacemaker that sends electrical signals to the muscle, causing it to contract rhythmically, which churns the food up to mix and digest it.

How long does food stay in the stomach?

About 1–3 hours. Fluids spend less time there, but fatty foods delay the emptying of the stomach so that whatever was eaten with them will get held back for longer as well.

How much digestive juice does the stomach produce?

The stomach produces 2–3 litres (4–6 pints) of gastric juice each day. This contains hydrochloric acid, which can make the contents of the stomach very acid. You may hear healthcare professionals talking about the 'pH' of your stomach. A neutral pH is 7, with numbers bigger than this meaning alkaline, and smaller numbers meaning acid – the pH of your stomach can be as low as 1! The function of the acid is to help digest protein and to protect against infection by killing any bacteria ingested with the food. Surprisingly, reducing acid production with medicines, surgery or disease seems to make remarkably little difference to a person's health. Gastric juice also contains enzymes; the main function of these is to digest protein.

What can go wrong with the stomach?

Ulcers in the stomach usually produce pain in the upper abdomen that is related to food. They are mostly caused by an infection acquired in childhood with a bacterium called *Helicobacter pylori* (*H. pylori*) or from taking non-steroidal anti-inflammatory drugs (NSAIDs) such as aspirin, ibuprofen, naproxen and many others. Ulcers associated with NSAIDs are painless in at least half the people who have them.

Cancer of the stomach is rare under the age of 50 years. It presents with upper abdominal pain, vomiting, weight loss or anaemia (a low level of iron in the blood). It is caused by *H. pylori* infection and environmental factors. Stomach cancer is very common in Japan where the diet is high in salt- and nitrate-containing foods such as dried fish, pickles and processed meats. Interestingly, Japanese people who adopt a Western diet reduce their risk of stomach cancer.

Problems with the movements of the stomach (dysmotility) are caused by poor co-ordination of the stomach muscles. This is one of the most common causes of indigestion. Typical symptoms include feeling full early on in a meal, a feeling of fullness and bloating in the upper abdomen, reflux, and upper abdominal pain that responds poorly to acid-reducing medicines. Dysmotility is fairly common in patients with IBS.

What is a hiatus hernia? My friend suggested it could explain my problems.

As we said earlier, the chest and the abdomen are separated by the diaphragm. It has an opening in its centre through which the oesophagus passes to empty into the stomach. In a hiatus hernia, part of the upper part of the stomach is shifted up through this opening and into the chest. A hiatus hernia is not visible from the outside. Its significance is that it allows more acid to reflux up into the oesophagus. The usual symptom is 'heartburn', although acid in the oesophagus can also cause pain in the upper abdomen. The medical treatment is medication to reduce acid production by the stomach. Self-treatment involves weight loss, stopping smoking, and drinking less alcohol and coffee.

THE DUODENUM

The duodenum is the first 25 centimetres (10 inches) of the small bowel (Figure 1.1) and has a diameter of 4–5 centimetres (2 inches). It curves in a C shape around the head of the pancreas. The pancreatic duct and the bile duct (from the gall bladder) join to empty into the duodenum. The pancreas and gall bladder produce substances that help to break down the food (sugars, proteins and fats, respectively) so that it can be digested.

What can go wrong with the duodenum?

The acidic contents of the stomach empty into the duodenum, so it may become inflamed and ulcerated. Duodenal ulcers cause pain in the upper abdomen, and sometimes back pain that is related to food, or even occasionally relieved by food. As with stomach ulcers, infection with the bacterium *H. pylori* and taking NSAIDs are the predominant causes.

Cancer of the duodenum is very rare.

THE SMALL BOWEL

The small intestine, or small bowel, is made up of the jejunum (the upper half) and the ileum (the lower half; Figure 1.1). There is no sharp distinction between them, and it's just convention to call the parts this. The length of the small bowel varies from 3 to 10 metres (10–33 feet), the average length being 6 metres (24 feet). It tapers from about 3 centimetres down to about 2 centimetres (1 inch) in width.

The time taken for food to pass through the small bowel varies from about 2 to 6 hours, with an average of about 3.5 hours. Air can be propelled though the small bowel much more quickly, and swallowed air may reach the anus within half an hour.

The small intestine is one of the most important organs in the body. Most of the digestion and absorption of the food occurs here. Life without a small intestine is difficult and needs food solutions to be infused directly into the bloodstream. This is called total parenteral nutrition; in the long term, it is invariably complicated by serious infections. Transplantation of the small bowel is only in its early days and can't yet be used to solve this problem.

What can go wrong with the small intestine?

The small intestine needs to absorb about 9 litres (18 pints) of fluid every day. This is made up of about 1.5 litres that has been taken in with the food and about 7.5 litres secreted as digestive juices. If the small intestine doesn't do this, the consequence is severe diarrhoea with rapid dehydration. Small bowel dysfunction occurs with infection, coeliac disease and Crohn's disease (see Chapter 8 for more on this).

It was once thought that the small bowel was not involved in IBS. However, recent evidence convincingly shows that abdominal bloating is predominantly due to air that has been retained in the small bowel.

The small bowel is almost sterile, normally containing few if any bacteria. In some people, bacteria from the large bowel manage to pass back up into the small bowel. These usually get flushed out, but if they manage to take hold, we get a condition called 'small bowel bacterial overgrowth'. These bacteria then interfere with the digestion and absorption of the food. The symptoms that result can be similar to those seen in IBS. In fact, small bowel bacterial overgrowth has been suggested as a cause of IBS (see Chapters 3 and 8).

Cancer of the small bowel is very rare.

THE LARGE BOWEL

The large intestine varies in length, but is usually about 1–1.5 metres (5 feet) long and about 5 centimetres (2 inches) wide. There is a valve between the small bowel and the large bowel called the ileo-caecal valve, which to some extent prevents backflow. The different parts of the large bowel are given their own names (caecum, ascending colon, transverse colon, descending colon, sigmoid colon; see Figure 1.1), but there are really no distinct divisions between them.

The large bowel acts to absorb about 1 litre (2 pints) from the mixture that pours in from the small bowel. This is because a more solid formed stool is easier to hold until we are ready to defecate. It normally takes 24–48 hours for food residue to pass through the large bowel, but gas is conducted much faster and can reach the anus within half an hour.

The large bowel is full of bacteria; indeed, half of the stool that we pass is made up of bacterial cell bodies. It is therefore not surprising that antibiotics disturb bowel function, usually leading to diarrhoea.

What can go wrong with the large bowel?

Compared with our other organs, the large bowel is relatively unimportant. You can easily live without part or all of it, and many people indeed do just that because large bowel problems are common.

Infective diarrhoea caused by viruses or bacteria is common in the large bowel. When the rectum becomes inflamed, from whatever cause, we feel an urgent call to stool whenever anything enters it – liquid, solid or gas. But because the large bowel is required to absorb only about a litre of fluid a day, fluid loss is minimal compared with small bowel dysfunction and rarely causes severe dehydration. Large bowel dysfunction is therefore usually associated with frequent, small-volume, loose stools.

Cancer of the large bowel affects about 1 in 25 people, presenting as a change in bowel habit to loose stools, bleeding or anaemia. It is rare under the age of 50 and is often cured by surgical resection.

Diverticular disease is increasingly common as we get older, affecting up to 60% of 60-year-olds. In many people, diverticular disease causes no problems at all. In others, it is associated with left-sided spasmodic pains and a change in bowel habit that cannot be distinguished from that of IBS. In a few people, diverticular disease produces more serious complications such as bleeding and infections.

Inflammatory bowel disease is a consequence of an overactive immune system in the bowel. It causes inflammation not related to infection, which damages the bowel. This shows up as diarrhoea, usually with blood. There are several 'inflammatory bowel diseases', as they are called, but ulcerative colitis and Crohn's disease are the most common. In their milder forms, they can be mistaken for IBS, but IBS does not develop into Crohn's disease or ulcerative colitis. Conversely, however, many people with inflammatory bowel disease will go on to also develop IBS.

Although bloating is now recognised to be mainly a consequence of problems in the small bowel, most of the other symptoms of IBS are thought to arise largely from the large bowel.

THE RECTUM, ANAL CANAL AND ANUS

The lowermost part of the large bowel is designed to keep a person continent, that is, stop the faeces leaking out when we don't want them to. The rectum (see Figure 1.1) is 12–15 centimetres (about 5–6 inches) long. It is named from the Latin word *regere* meaning 'to straighten, correct or rule', but although the rectum is straight in some mammals, in humans it is actually curved along the sacrum and attaches to the anal canal at an angle of 80–90 degrees.

Contrary to popular belief, the rectum is not a storage area for the stool but is usually empty. It is more sensitive to distension than other parts of the large bowel and can detect a volume as low as 80–120 ml (a small cupful). At larger volumes, for example 200–300 ml, the sensation of pressure in the rectum is greater, leading to an increasingly strong urge to defecate. In most people, the urge to defecate is usually irresistible at a rectal volume of over 400 ml. These volumes vary between individuals, however, and fall with age. In people with IBS, the rectum is more sensitive to distension. This partly explains why they have to rush to the toilet more frequently just to pass small amounts of stool or fluid.

My doctor mentioned the pubo-rectalis muscle. What is this?

The pubo-rectalis is one of the muscles in the pelvis. It runs from the pubic bones at the front, towards the back, around the lower end of the rectum, and back to the pubic bone (Figure 1.2). So it acts as a sling, pulling the rectum forward to create an 80–90 degree angle between the rectum and the anal canal. When we defecate, the pubo-rectalis muscle relaxes, allowing this angle to straighten out so that the stool can pass out more easily.

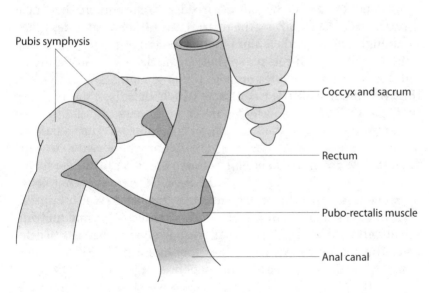

Pubis symphysis

Coccyx and sacrum

Rectum

Pubo-rectalis muscle

Anal canal

Figure 1.2 The pubo-rectalis sling.

I've always been a bit embarrassed to ask, but what happens when we defecate?

The anal canal is normally held tightly shut by the muscle bands that encircle it. These are called the anal sphincters. When the rectum is distended by stool or gas passing down from the colon, the internal sphincter (the upper one) relaxes slightly, allowing some of the rectal contents to pass into the anal canal.

The lining of the anal canal is very sensitive and can detect the difference between solid, liquid and gas. If it detects gas, the anal sphincters usually relax even more, allowing the gas to escape as flatulence. Liquid in the anal canal usually leads to a desperate desire to defecate, which has to be countered by a conscious effort to tighten the anal sphincter. When the anal canal detects solid matter, it gives us a choice: settle down to defecate, or contract the anal sphincters strongly, pushing the faeces back into the rectum until it is more convenient for us to go to the toilet.

To defecate, we sit or squat in order to straighten the angle between the anal canal and the rectum. An earlier answer described how this angle is partly maintained by a band of muscle called the pubo-rectalis, which relaxes so that the angle can be straightened out. The rectum now lines up with the anal canal. The muscles in the abdominal wall then contract, which increases the pressure within the abdomen and forces the stool to pass out of the large bowel.

Does it do any harm to put off going to the toilet?

Most of us resist the urge to defecate, the 'call to stool', every so often for social convenience. This is perfectly normal and will do no harm. But doing this regularly will lessen the message to defecate. The rectum can then become more tolerant of large volumes, which is a common cause of constipation.

Sometimes I need to rush to the toilet to pass a stool soon after eating or even during the meal. Is the food passing right through me that quickly?

You are actually describing a prominent gastrocolic reflex. A reflex is an unconscious automatic response in which stimulation of one part of the body results in activity in another. For example, tapping the tendon under the knee leads to reflex contraction of the thigh muscle. In the gut, filling and distension of the stomach leads to nervous impulses that stimulate activity in the bowel. This is a normal reflex. It is stronger in some people than others, and it is often more prominent in IBS and inflammatory bowel disease.

The simplest way of controlling it is to eat smaller meals, or to eat more slowly so as to reduce the distension of the stomach. Eating less fat may help too. Fatty foods tend to slow emptying of the stomach, so a fatty meal will tend to distend the stomach more. You may also wish to avoid taking caffeine with your meal as it will increase the stimulation of your bowel.

SUMMARY

- ◼ The gastrointestinal tract is basically a long tube from the mouth to the anus.

- ◼ Food normally spends about 1–3 hours in the stomach, 2–6 hours in the small bowel and 24–48 hours in the large bowel.

- ◼ Gas, such as swallowed air, will pass through much more quickly and may reach the anus within half an hour.

- ◼ The small bowel is the most important organ of digestion but, compared with other organs, it is rarely involved in disease.

- ◼ The small bowel is virtually sterile; any bacteria that enter it are flushed out into the large bowel.

- ◼ The large bowel is full of bacteria.

■ The large bowel collects undigested food, solidifies it by absorbing excess water and holds it until we defecate.

■ Although the large bowel is, compared with the small bowel, relatively unimportant, it is a common cause of disease.

■ The most common large bowel problem is IBS. The most serious problem is large bowel cancer.

2 | Epidemiology – who gets IBS?

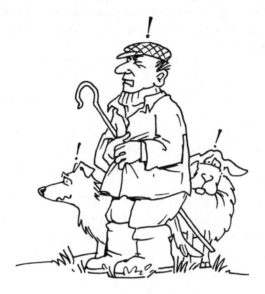

Epidemiology is the study of how often medical conditions occur in different groups of people. It characterises the condition in terms of age, sex, lifestyle habits, social and economic behaviours, ethnic origin and association with other diseases, conditions or treatments. This information is intended to give us clues to the cause of the condition and to suggest treatments or preventive strategies.

Can you define the irritable bowel syndrome in one sentence?

In irritable bowel syndrome (IBS), the function of the bowel is disturbed, causing symptoms, but its structure is normal.

How common is irritable bowel syndrome?

The individual symptoms that constitute IBS – constipation, diarrhoea, bloating and abdominal pain – are so common that most of us can expect to experience them at some time. It's when they come together, persist and interfere with daily life that we begin to feel that something is wrong. This constellation of bowel symptoms has come to be known as IBS, having previously been known in different guises as an irritable or spastic colon.

Depending on the criteria used to define IBS, about 9–23% of the world population are affected. In the UK, about 4-6% of the population have been given a formal diagnosis of IBS, but surveys suggest that a further 8% have undiagnosed IBS. In other words, at least 1 in 10 people have IBS to some extent. It is the most common gastroenterological problem seen by family doctors even though many people never go to the doctor with their IBS symptoms, so a formal diagnosis is never made.

If you have had symptoms for over a year without a recent change, without unintended weight loss or blood in the stool, there is no need to see your doctor for a 'formal' diagnosis of IBS. Many people come to terms with their symptoms of IBS, learn to live with them and lead perfectly normal lives.

LIFE FACTORS

We're always being told our Western lifestyle is unhealthy.
Is IBS predominantly a disease of Western developed countries?

IBS is not just related to modern living or the lifestyle of developed countries. It exists in every society that has been examined. The number of people said to be affected varies from 3.5% in Iran to 30% in Nigeria. These differences probably, at least partly, reflect the criteria used to diagnose IBS, how the questions about it were posed and cultural differences in answering them. Interestingly, the balance between constipation-predominant and diarrhoea-predominant IBS also varies. Constipation is said to dominate in Bangladesh and Singapore, whereas diarrhoea is more common in parts of China and India.

Is IBS more common in women?

IBS appears to be at least twice as common in women than in men. In one survey, 86% of people with IBS attending their family doctor in the UK were women. The reason for this is unknown. In a few countries (India, Sri Lanka and Japan, for example), IBS isn't more common in women. This may be because Asian men are more likely than Asian women to tell their doctor about symptoms that could be caused by IBS. Since the diagnosis of IBS depends entirely on people describing their symptoms, cultural issues may contribute to the number of men and women being diagnosed. British men are notoriously reluctant to talk about bodily functions, and this may partly explain why more women than men in the UK appear to have IBS.

I'm sure my IBS is worse during my period. Is IBS affected by menstruation?

Many women report that their IBS symptoms are worse during their periods. Occasionally, they feel their symptoms are worse in the middle of the cycle. It is possible that these changes in severity relate to changes in the levels of the hormones oestrogen and progesterone.

Oestrogen levels are highest near the mid-point of the cycle, and in women without IBS, the stools tend to be firmer at this time. When oestrogen and progesterone levels fall towards the end of the cycle, the lining of the uterus breaks down and menstruation starts. In women without IBS, we know that the stools tend to be somewhat looser and more frequent during menstruation. These effects may be exacerbated in women with IBS, so that diarrhoea is worse during menstruation and constipation is worse between periods.

Interestingly, a recent study has suggested that the rectum becomes more sensitive to distension in women with IBS during menstruation, which would explain an increase in pain. Alternatively, some women may find menstruation stressful anyway, so that other symptoms can become less tolerable.

I've just been put on hormone replacement therapy (HRT).
Does HRT affect IBS?

There is just one study suggesting that women with IBS have less bloating when they take HRT, but it doesn't seem to affect other symptoms. IBS is not a reason to try HRT.

I've got IBS and I'm worried that my son will get it too. Is there a
genetic influence?

One way of assessing the heritability of a condition is to look at how often the disease occurs in *both* members of a pair of twins. This is called the concordance rate. Both twins are assumed to have had the same environmental influences, but identical twins have all their genes in common, whereas non-identical twins have about half their genes in common. Therefore, if genes are important in the aetiology of a disease, that is, in what causes the disease, the concordance rate will be higher in identical twins.

One study of twins has shown a concordance rate of 33% for IBS in identical twins compared with just 13% for non-identical twins. This suggests that genetic influences *are* important. Although no specific gene has been identified, a recent study has demonstrated an association between certain forms of the gene coding for a protein that transports a substance called serotonin (which affects the movement of the gut) and diarrhoea-predominant IBS. Hopefully, as we discover more information on the human genome, we will better understand how different genes interact with the environment to produce illnesses.

How old are people when they develop IBS?

In a European survey of over 40 000 people published in 2003, symptoms that could be explained by IBS were found in 12.2% of 18–34-year-olds, 9.9% of 35–54-year-olds and 7% of over 55-year-olds. Similar results were found in an American study.

IBS seems to be most common in young women but exists in all age groups.

How often will the average family doctor see a new case of IBS?

Large surveys from the UK and USA have estimated that about 2–4 new cases of IBS occur for each 1000 people and are diagnosed by family doctors every year. As the average family doctor in the UK has about 2000 patients, he or she will see 4–8 new cases of IBS each year. As there is no cure for IBS, many patients will see their doctor again and again. It has been estimated that 1 in 12 of family doctor consultations in the UK are to do with gastroenterological problems. About a third of these patients will be asking about symptoms related to IBS, so that IBS is probably the most common gastroenterological problem seen by family doctors.

Although family doctors probably refer only about a third of the patients they see with IBS for a specialist opinion, IBS may form up to 40% of a hospital gastroenterologist's outpatient practice.

Is smoking linked to IBS?

Smoking has not been linked to IBS. However, it is known to exacerbate Crohn's disease, even though it may actually help ulcerative colitis.

Is alcohol linked to IBS?

Excess alcohol consumption tends to make the stools looser and is in some people a cause of diarrhoea. Nausea, vomiting and pain in the upper abdomen are also frequently associated with excess alcohol, or with alcohol withdrawal. Alcohol consumption is not, however, associated with IBS.

IBS AND OTHER CONDITIONS

What about obesity? It's always on the TV and in the papers about how obesity is rising. Is IBS associated with this?

There is no association between IBS and obesity; obesity does not cause IBS. Losing weight can cure some cases of heartburn and indigestion, such as from acid reflux from the stomach, but it will not improve IBS.

Is IBS more common after a hysterectomy or any other operation?

In a study of over 40 000 European women, hysterectomy (removal of the womb) was not associated with IBS. There was a slightly higher rate of previous appendectomy (removal of the appendix) in IBS sufferers. This might be because both conditions cause pain in the right lower corner of the abdomen, so the IBS in these cases may initially have been mistaken for, for example, appendicitis. The rates of gall bladder, ovarian or bladder surgery were no higher in people with IBS.

I'd had bad gastroenteritis not long before I got IBS. Is IBS more common after a bout of gastroenteritis?

IBS occurring after gastroenteritis probably accounts for at least 10% of all cases of IBS. The risk of getting IBS following gastroen-teritis has been estimated to be 4–7% (4–7 people in every 100) in the year after the infection. This compares with an average risk in the general population of 0.2% (2 in a 1000) each year.

Is IBS more common after taking antibiotics?

This is something that some patients notice, but surveys haven't supported the idea. Antibiotic treatment frequently causes a loosening of the stool or actual diarrhoea because many of the bacteria that normally live in the large bowel are killed. This is not IBS, and the bowel habit usually returns to normal once the antibiotic treatment has been completed and the bowel's population of bacteria returns to normal.

Is IBS associated with indigestion?

In a study of over 40 000 Europeans, indigestion (dyspepsia), including gastro-oesophageal reflux (reflux of acid back from the stomach into the oesophagus) and peptic ulcer disease, was more common in those with IBS. In clinical practice, between a third and a half of people coming to the clinic with IBS-type symptoms will also describe symptoms of indigestion. Most of these people will not have ulcers or severe inflammation of their oesophagus (oesophagitis). Rather, they tend to have dysmotility (a lack of co-ordination of the stomach muscles) or mild acid reflux from the stomach into the oesophagus.

The relationship between indigestion and IBS is not surprising as stomach function can affect bowel function and vice versa. Filling of the stomach promotes muscular activity and emptying of the bowel. This is called the gastrocolic reflex, and it explains why people sometimes need to empty their bowel immediately after or even during a meal. Conversely, constipation slows down the emptying of partly digested food from the stomach, and it is easy to understand how severe constipation can produce symptoms of indigestion, nausea and vomiting.

Will having IBS mean I'll get cancer later?

No. IBS does not predispose to cancer or to any other serious disorder.

THE FUTURE

What is the prognosis for IBS? And how long does it last?

The symptoms of IBS usually come and go, so that people can have long-lasting periods when they hardly notice they have it.

In one study, fewer than a third of people were free of symptoms after 2 years, and in another, 1 in 20 people were free of symptoms after 5 years. IBS occurring after a bout of gastroenteritis (post-infectious IBS) may have a better prognosis – about 40% of people with this appear to recover after 5–6 years.

There is no cure for IBS, but you can rest assured that nothing more serious will develop from it. The symptoms of IBS do, however, tend to persist over the years. There is a lot you can do to make sure that they interfere as little as possible with your everyday life, and the aim of this book is to empower you to do so.

SUMMARY

■ IBS is very common, affecting about 10% of people of both sexes in all age groups and in all ethnicities and cultures.

■ The usual suspects – smoking, alcohol, obesity and a Western lifestyle – are not to blame.

3 | What causes IBS?

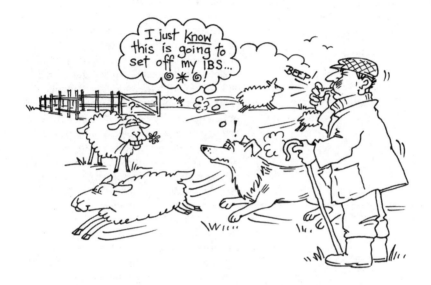

A syndrome is a collection of symptoms and signs that tend to occur and run together, producing a recognisable ailment. It may have a variety of causes or no definable cause. That's how it is with the irritable bowel syndrome (IBS). Many different causes have been suggested, but none has fully explained the many features that constitute IBS. As with other medical syndromes, it's possible for different aetiologies (causes) to produce the same symptoms. Many diseases arise through a combination of genetic, environmental and sometimes psychological factors, and this is likely to be the case with IBS.

Any theory that seeks to explain IBS must explain its key features (Table 3.1), and this chapter will outline some of the explanations that have been proposed for IBS.

Table 3.1 Key features of irritable bowel syndrome (IBS)

Key features of IBS	Comment
Common across all age groups, and ethnic groups	Most people will have some bowel symptoms at some time in their life
Psychological problems	Psychological factors such as anxiety or depression greatly exacerbate the symptoms of IBS, while IBS can also cause or exacerbate anxiety and depression. In general, people with IBS do not have an excess of mental health problems compared with the general population; many people with IBS don't have any psychological problems. Understandably, however, people with IBS who are also depressed and anxious will have more trouble coping with their symptoms and are more likely to see their doctor
Variability of symptoms	Not only can IBS produce opposite symptoms such as constipation or diarrhoea, but the nature of a person's symptoms can also change with time. Diarrhoea-predominant IBS can change to an alternating pattern or even to constipation, and vice versa
Variability over time	IBS comes and goes, sometimes over hours or days, sometimes over days, weeks or months
Lack of obvious physical or biochemical abnormalities	Most diseases are characterised by physical or biochemical abnormalities that we can find during a medical examination or test. In IBS, symptoms predominate, and medical tests of structure and function are normal

IS IBS A PSYCHOLOGICAL DISORDER?

Up to half of people seen in hospital clinics with IBS will have some form of psychological disturbance such as depression or anxiety. This may mean that psychological problems cause or exacerbate IBS, but equally it could simply mean that severe IBS causes or exacerbates psychological problems. Alternatively, the apparent association between psychological problems and IBS seen in hospital clinics may just be a result of the type of person that family doctors refer.

Both IBS and psychological problems are common. Understandably, the combination is more difficult to cope with, and people with IBS who are also depressed or anxious are more likely to consult their family doctor. The family doctor probably refers only about half of his or her patients with IBS to a hospital gastroenterologist. Not surprisingly, people with psychological problems in addition to IBS may not respond as well to simple measures or reassurance, so are more likely to be referred for a specialist opinion. Consequently, a large proportion of people who have been referred will have a psychological problem, including depression, anxiety, obsession or even a history of sexual or physical abuse. There is therefore a widespread belief that IBS has a psychological origin.

But when individuals with IBS in the general population are examined, they probably have no more psychological problems than do the rest of the general population. It is perfectly understandable that people with psychological problems, stress or anxiety are more likely to seek medical attention. Moreover, stress will make any illness worse. So although IBS is not primarily a psychological disorder, it does have psychological components, which should not be ignored and which can be treated so that individuals with IBS can gain control over their condition.

So some people with IBS have psychological problems. What does this mean for me?

The primary cause of IBS may not be a psychological illness. Yet there is often an important psychological element that exacerbates and prolongs the problems and makes the symptoms more difficult to deal with. You should consider whether you have any problems or stresses that might be associated with your IBS symptoms.

CANDIDA SYNDROME – YEAST INFECTION OR HYPERSENSITIVITY?

What is Candida?

There are three major groups of fungi: moulds, yeasts and mushrooms. *Candida* is a yeast that exists as a one-celled organism somewhat larger than a bacterium. Like other yeasts, *Candida* is able to ferment carbohydrates to alcohol – just like yeasts do in beer-making.

So am I likely to have Candida *living in my body?*

Candida can be cultured from the faeces in up to 80% of healthy adults. It is regarded as part of the normal flora (the bacteria usually present) of the skin, mouth, intestine and vagina.

Does Candida *cause disease?*

The number of *Candida* organisms is usually controlled by competition with the bacteria already present. Following treatment with antibiotics, these bacteria decrease in number and the number of *Candida* organisms increases. This can show up as the condition called thrush.

Thrush appears as whitish, velvety plaques in the mouth and on the tongue, or in and around the vagina. Under this whitish material is red tissue that may bleed. The lesions can slowly increase in both number and size. Treatment that suppresses the immune system with corticosteroids can also be complicated by thrush. Treatment for *Candida* is usually straightforward, with nystatin or other antifungal drugs.

A friend mentioned 'Candida syndrome' to me. What is this?

The idea of the Candida syndrome was suggested and popularised by William Crook in his book *The Yeast Connection*. It has excited much attention in the popular press but very little interest in academic circles. Other names given to this presumed condition include *Candida*-related complex, polysystemic candidiasis and chronic candidiasis.

The theory goes as follows. The components of our modern lifestyle, including antibiotics, oral contraceptives and diets rich in yeast-containing foods or readily utilisable carbohydrates, mean that when *Candida* colonises a person's intestine, it starts to overgrow. This overgrowth results in a variety of symptoms, for example chronic fatigue, anxiety and depression, headaches and respiratory symptoms, as well as an irritable bowel.

Can Candida syndrome be treated?

Yes. Treatment involves long-term therapy with antifungal agents at increasing doses until the symptoms resolve. Oral (by mouth) as well as vaginal nystatin is recommended. Other potent antifungal medicines such as ketoconazole have also been used. Modifying the diet, including restricting sugar and other simple carbohydrates, is used to limit the nutrients that the *Candida* needs.

But is there any evidence that Candida syndrome actually exists?

There are a number of small scientific trials of treatment for *Candida* that show an improvement in symptoms such as diarrhoea and flatulence, but these are difficult to interpret as they did not include any controls.

(Because some conditions get better without specific treatment, and because people sometimes get better simply because they 'believe' in the treatment they are getting, any treatment must be compared against another treatment, usually a placebo – an inert substance given as a medicine for its suggestive effect – to know whether it really works. In scientific studies, the 'other' treatment is called the control. Studies without controls are of limited value because we cannot know whether the person's condition has improved because of the treatment, because it was going to improve anyway, or because the person believed it was going to improve.)

In one trial, nystatin was used to treat women with recurring vaginal thrush and many other symptoms consistent with *Candida* syndrome. The treatment cured the thrush but had no effect on the other symptoms, implying that these 'other' symptoms had nothing to do with the *Candida* infection. Similarly, a study published in the prestigious *New England Journal of Medicine* concluded that when women presumed to have candidiasis hypersensitivity syndrome took nystatin, their bodily and psychological symptoms did not improve significantly more than they did with a placebo (a dummy treatment). Treatment with nystatin therefore appears to be unwarranted and ineffective for IBS or chronic fatigue-type symptoms.

Should I try nystatin anyway? What have I got to lose?

Nystatin is relatively inexpensive and safe. It can cause gastrointestinal side effects such as nausea, vomiting and diarrhoea, and occasional allergic reactions. More potent antifungal drugs such as fluconazole are much more expensive and more likely to have side effects. Moreover, most '*Candida* therapists' also recommend a diet low in sugar and simple carbohydrates to reduce the proliferation of *Candida* in the gut, along with the nystatin; they tend too to suggest various supplements and probiotics to enhance the growth of the natural bacteria in the gut.

The more you look into it, the more complicated and expensive the treatment for this so-called syndrome becomes. The proponents of these treatments employ an evangelist approach, and if you believe them you may well benefit from a 'placebo response' (see Chapter 12). As the placebo response can last for 3 months, this may be worthwhile for you, but I suggest you direct your energy instead towards treatments that have a more scientific basis.

Why are doctors so sceptical of the Candida syndrome as a cause of IBS?

Both hospital doctors and family doctors see *Candida* infections fairly frequently, but we don't associate them with IBS. Nor do we notice any improvement in pre-existing IBS if an incidental *Candida* infection is treated.

Overgrowth of *Candida* occurs in the mouth or the vagina of perfectly healthy people. It is unpleasant but easily treated. More serious infections with *Candida* affecting the lungs, oesophagus, liver, blood and other organs are not unusual in people with a weak immune system. Some of these patients will have IBS – because it is a common condition. In my experience, however, they do not complain of new or more severe IBS symptoms in association with an obvious overgrowth of *Candida*. Moreover, although powerful antifungal treatment usually resolves their *Candida* overgrowth, the IBS remains.

SMALL BOWEL BACTERIAL OVERGROWTH

What is small bowel bacterial overgrowth?

This is a syndrome in which excessive numbers of bacteria in the small bowel interfere with the digestion and absorption of the food, causing diarrhoea. There may also be bloating, wind and weight loss.

The small bowel, where most of our digestion and absorption takes place, is normally almost sterile. It harbours very few bacteria.

By contrast, the large bowel is full of bacteria, so that half the content of the stool is made up of bacteria!

There are a number of mechanisms that keep the small bowel free of bacteria. Acid in the stomach kills most of the bacteria that we ingest with our food. The continuous, rapid movement through the small bowel prevents stagnant pools of nutrients where bacteria could breed, and clears away any bacteria that have migrated up from the large bowel. There is also a valve between the small bowel and the large bowel – the ileocaecal valve – that limits backflow.

But these mechanisms may fail, allowing bacteria to enter and multiply within the small bowel. Surprisingly, the bacteria do not actually invade the body from the small bowel, so there are no symptoms of infection. People with small bowel bacterial overgrowth do not usually feel unwell and do not have a fever. They usually come to the doctor with diarrhoea, which can be watery or fatty, and they may just feel that they have an irritable bowel.

Who gets small bowel bacterial overgrowth?

Anyone can get this disorder, but some people are more likely to. Older people produce less acid to sterilise their food, their immune system may be weaker and the movement in their small bowel may not be as co-ordinated. In those who have diabetes, those who have had surgery on their small bowel and those who have nerve damage, the movement of the small bowel may be abnormal, leading to stagnation, which allows bacteria to multiply.

Is small bowel bacterial overgrowth likely to have caused my IBS?

The symptoms of small bowel bacterial overgrowth can be identical to those of IBS, particularly diarrhoea-predominant IBS. Bloating and diarrhoea are prominent in both syndromes.

One American study of 111 patients with IBS found evidence of small bowel bacterial overgrowth in 93 (84%) of the patients. Half the patients were treated with an antibiotic and half with a placebo (a dummy medicine). About a third (35%) of the patients receiving the antibiotic improved, compared with 11% of those who had received the placebo. Although this study has not been repeated, it does suggest that at least a proportion of patients with IBS have small bowel bacterial overgrowth and will respond to treatment with antibiotics.

Does this theory have any limitations as an explanation for IBS?

It is difficult to understand how small bowel bacterial overgrowth can cause constipation as well as diarrhoea. It has been suggested that some patients have bacteria that produce methane gas, and that the methane may slow the bowel down. Evidence for this effect of methane is sparse at present, so the explanation is unconvincing. Moreover, most people with IBS have pain as a significant component of their symptoms, whereas most patients with small bowel bacterial overgrowth do not have pain, or if they do, it is not a major feature. Furthermore, small bowel bacterial overgrowth affects men and women equally, whereas IBS is probably far more common in women.

It is unlikely therefore that this condition explains IBS. But it may be part of the problem in people with IBS who have predominant diarrhoea. I frequently treat patients with otherwise unexplained diarrhoea and bloating with antibiotics. In elderly patients, those with diabetes or those who have had surgery on their bowel or stomach, this is often the first therapeutic approach. And a proportion of patients do show a benefit, making the treatment worthwhile.

What does small bowel bacterial overgrowth mean for me? Should I ask my doctor for an antibiotic?

If your main problem is diarrhoea, and if it cannot be easily controlled by low doses of loperamide or similar medications that slow the bowel down, then small bowel bacterial overgrowth is possible. It is particularly common in those with diabetes, people who have had abdominal surgery and the elderly. In such circumstances, it is reasonable to ask your doctor for a course of an antibiotic such as metronidazole.

FOOD ALLERGY AND INTOLERANCE

Is it possible to eliminate the symptoms of IBS by avoiding specific foods? A large proportion of people with IBS believe their symptoms are an adverse reaction to food and might like to try this approach (see Chapter 10).

It is undeniable that eating certain foods increases the severity of symptoms for many people. What is not clear is whether the food causes the symptoms or just exacerbates them. Does food allergy and intolerance cause IBS, or are these different problems with exactly the same symptoms? Is it possible to eliminate the symptoms of IBS simply by avoiding certain foods? – the question remains controversial.

Reactions that are classed as allergic are caused by a response of the immune system to a specific foreign (that is, something that is not part of the body) protein. Intolerance, however, does not happen through the immune system. The mechanisms of intolerance to some foods, such as lactose, are well worked out. For other foods, such as wheat, they are not. I expect too that other intolerances are still waiting to be discovered.

Although some people with IBS symptoms can gain enormous benefit from avoiding certain foods such as dairy or wheat products, others struggle with food diaries and different diets without any results. They discover after much effort that their response to different foods is too inconsistent to draw any conclusions.

To guide individuals on which foods to avoid, a more recent approach has involved identifying a particular type of antibody, called IgG antibody, to specific foods. These IgG antibodies circulate in the blood and help to protect us against bacterial and viral infections. They represent an immune reaction to a current or previous invading organism. The assumption is that if an IgG antibody to a food exists in someone's blood, the person may be allergic to that food. A diet avoiding all the foods to which a person has IgG antibodies would logically, therefore, eliminate any symptoms arising from food allergies.

But this is a controversial theory because it is *IgE* antibodies that mediate allergy, and the presence of IgG antibodies to food has not previously been thought of as significant. Moreover, people can have IgG antibodies to many different foods, and a diet designed to eliminate all these foods is likely to be difficult to follow and may not be nutritionally balanced. Despite that, a recent study showed that, of the people who managed to stick to such individualised diets, 50% experienced a significant improvement in their symptoms.

What are the limitations of food allergy and intolerance as an explanation for IBS?

Most allergic or intolerant reactions are associated with diarrhoea rather than constipation, and at least a third of people with IBS have predominant constipation. Food allergy does not address the variability in symptoms either between people or in the same person over time. Nor does it address the psychological aspects of IBS and its relationship to stress.

So what does it mean for me? Is it worth avoiding certain foods?

A dietary approach will work for some people, some of the time, to a certain extent. Certainly, if you discover specific foods that consistently cause you problems, you can avoid them, or decide to eat them despite the symptoms. But you need to be aware that some people are drawn into investing a lot of time and effort in trying a dietary approach to IBS. They can become a little obsessed with avoiding food that might have a detrimental effect on their health in general and on their personal relationships.

There *are* dietary approaches that are worth trying (see Chapter 10), but if they fail to produce significant benefit, it is better to accept that the symptoms reflect the reaction of the gut to foods in general rather than specific items in the diet. We should probably agree with the American author Mark Twain: 'Eat what you like, and let the food fight it out inside.'

INFLAMMATION IN THE BOWEL

I've got IBS. Does this mean that my bowel is inflamed?

Pathologists examining samples of tissue (biopsy specimens) taken from the bowel are unable to differentiate between biopsies from people with and without IBS. Even the 'healthy' bowel is in a constant state of mild inflammation as the immune system battles to control the organisms that normally live in the gut. There may be no obvious extra gut inflammation in those who have IBS, but this does not rule out an increase, too small to be seen under the microscope, in inflammatory cells that may start or contribute to the problem.

Do anti-inflammatory treatments work in IBS? Should I try aspirin, ibuprofen or even steroids?

The treatments that we use to control excess inflammation in inflammatory bowel disease (ulcerative colitis and Crohn's disease) do not improve IBS. Corticosteroids can initially cause a feeling of well-being in anyone who takes them, but other than that they are no help in IBS. Preparations of a medicine called mesalazine (brand names, for example, Asacol, Salofalk and Pentasa) which is used for inflammatory bowel disease are completely ineffective in IBS. Non-steroidal anti-inflammatory drugs (NSAIDs) such as aspirin, ibuprofen and diclofenac are very effective at controlling pain in the joints and inflamed soft tissues but are useless for IBS.

My IBS started after an infection. Does this make a difference?

About 10% of patients with IBS date the start of their problem to a bout of infective gastroenteritis. Infection with an organism called *Campylobacter* is particularly associated with subsequent IBS, usually diarrhoea predominant. In these people, there has been shown to be an excess of a type of white blood cell called a T-lymphocyte in the gut wall, which indicates persisting inflammation. This inflammation is likely to be associated with the production of chemical messengers such as prostaglandins and serotonin, which will increase intestinal secretions and muscular contraction; this then leads to diarrhoea. They may also increase the sensitivity of the bowel to stretching, causing pain.

Is it possible for a previous, unidentified infection to have caused my IBS?

It *is* possible for a previous, unidentified infection to change the character of the immune system in the gut. Our current methods may not be sensitive enough to detect changes in the immune system that might contribute to IBS symptoms. So the statement that only 10% of IBS arises after an infection may be an underestimate.

Could a change in the type of bacteria that inhabit the bowel result in symptoms of IBS?

Some supporters of the inflammation theory of IBS suggest that a change in the gut flora (the bacteria that inhabit the bowel), arising after infection or after treatment with antibiotics, may be important. More harmful bacteria may increase in number, and the immune response to this may lead to symptoms. Indeed, some IBS patients associate the start of their problem to treatment with antibiotics.

Is this where probiotics come in?

Probiotics are preparations of living organisms that are thought to be beneficial to health. They are bacteria such as *Lactobacillus* and bifidobacteria; when ingested in sufficient numbers, these manage to survive the upper gut to populate the large bowel. They may be beneficial by producing substances that increase the acidity of the large bowel so that it becomes a less appealing environment for more harmful bacteria. Moreover, they may help to stop harmful bacteria getting into the gut wall simply by their physical presence.

Treatment with probiotics is in its early days. A few studies have shown some benefit in IBS. Probiotics are commercially available in health food stores, and the idea of treating IBS with probiotics is attractive and generates great interest. However, there isn't yet enough clinical evidence to enable clear guidelines to be written. Large, well-designed, controlled clinical trials using specific probiotics are warranted.

How does gut inflammation fail to explain the features of IBS?

The inflammatory disorders of the intestine that we know about, such as ulcerative colitis and infections such as *Campylobacter* enteritis, almost always cause diarrhoea. But constipation is frequently a feature of IBS, and even people with diarrhoea-predominant IBS may have periods of constipation. Moreover, most inflammatory disorders respond to corticosteroids – often dramatically – whereas IBS does not. Gut infections are usually self-limiting and do not recur without a repeated exposure. By contrast, IBS will wax and wane in severity and goes on and on, or recurs for no apparent reason.

Finally, in inflammatory disorders in general, the severity of the symptoms is closely related to the severity of inflammation that we find in the affected organ. In IBS, however, we can see severe symptoms with minimal, if any, inflammation.

So is the gut inflamed in IBS or not? What are the implications for me?

We are not yet sure. The gut immune system may be altered in subtle ways that we cannot currently detect with any reliability. The current anti-inflammatory treatments that we use to suppress the immune system do not work for IBS. It may be that, as our understanding of the role of the immune system in IBS increases, new treatments will emerge. Probiotics might be the precursors of these treatments.

VISCERAL HYPERSENSITIVITY

Visceral hypersensitivity is a feature in most patients with IBS.

What is meant by 'visceral hypersensitivity'?

The word 'visceral' refers to the internal organs of the body, especially the intestine, as opposed to the skin, muscles and bone. 'Hypersensitivity' means an abnormally excessive response to normal stimuli. The concept of visceral hypersensitivity evolved in the 1980s to explain how people can get gastrointestinal symptoms without any apparent abnormality in the structure or function of their intestine.

We have sensory organs monitoring every part of our body, and most of these never generate any conscious perceptions. Most of the sensory signals play a role in the automatic regulation of digestion, and usually the only signals that are perceived consciously are those which require a response, for example a desire to defecate. The brain has mechanisms that prevent the vast majority of signals from our internal organs from reaching consciousness. It seems, however, that this mechanism may not work quite as well in some people. The result is visceral hypersensitivity.

This means that people with IBS are more sensitive than usual to events occurring within their intestine. These 'events' may simply be the normal contraction and relaxation of the bowel wall, or the normal exposure or reaction to food.

Does this problem only affect the organs inside the body?

It is not unusual to have odd sensations from various parts of the body. You may feel that your hand or your face is swollen or hot, or just different. You will then examine the offending part, feel it, look in the mirror and so on . . . . If this examination is entirely unremarkable, you will be reassured and most likely forget about the odd sensation.

Unfortunately, when we get odd sensations from the inside, we cannot check them out as easily, so they are more difficult to ignore. The anxiety we then feel may make us even more aware of sensations arising internally, which amplifies them still further.

So if I've got IBS, am I likely to have visceral hypersensitivity?

Visceral hypersensitivity is one of the most consistent findings in research studies on IBS. These studies mostly involve inflating a balloon in the rectum or lower bowel to determine the pressure or volume at which discomfort or pain is felt. Most people with IBS report discomfort or pain at significantly lower pressures or volumes, indicating that the bowel is more sensitive to stretching and pressure in IBS.

Do people with IBS have a lower pain threshold? Are they just more sensitive to pain?

No, people with IBS are not oversensitive. Pain thresholds are measured with graded electric shocks to the skin and are quite normal in people with IBS, even though they can be shown to have visceral sensitivity affecting the large bowel, the small bowel and even the oesophagus.

How and why, then, does visceral hypersensitivity happen?

There are sensors that respond to stretching, pressure or various chemicals located throughout the body, and report back to the brain. Most of the signals that these sensors generate never reach consciousness. The strength of the signal generated from a stimulus, such as increased pressure in a particular part of bowel, depends on a number of factors. Clearly, the stronger the stimulus, the greater the signal, but the strength of the signal also depends on the number of active sensors and their sensitivity to the stimulus.

Once the signal has been generated, it travels to the spinal cord, where it is altered. It may be either amplified or de-amplified. Nerve pathways from the brain also descend to the spinal cord and alter sensory transmission still further. Once the signal has reached the brain, it is changed yet again by nerve pathways from the brain's emotional centres. Thus, the increased pain signal that indicates visceral hypersensitivity can occur as a consequence of changes at several locations – the gut itself, the spinal cord or the brain – or indeed at all three sites.

What increases the pain signal from the gut?

Experiments have been performed on animals, mainly rats, to try to answer this question. They show that inflammation increases the sensitivity of the sensory nerves in the gut. The chemical signals that carry out the inflammatory response, such as prostaglandins, histamine and serotonin, also interact with the sensory mechanisms, increasing their sensitivity. This means that, for any stimulus, such as an increased pressure within a part of the bowel, a stronger signal is generated. The signal remains higher for up to 6 weeks after the inflammation has ended and healing has taken place.

People probably respond similarly to animals. It is common for an inflamed organ to be more sensitive, and to remain more sensitive for some time after healing. This is presumably an adaptive response to reduce the risk of re-injury. But it is unclear whether the increased sensitivity of the gut sensory mechanism persists for more than a few weeks in people, and to what extent it is responsible for the hypersensitivity of IBS. It is interesting that tricyclic antidepressants such as amitriptyline can directly affect nerve cells in animals to reduce their sensitivity, as in humans amitriptyline is one of the most successful drugs used to control IBS pain.

How is the pain signal modified in the spinal cord?

Nerves from our internal organs carrying pain signals initially go to the spinal cord. Here, the signal competes with other signals entering the cord before being transmitted upwards to the brain. Sensory signals will therefore compete with pain signals to reduce the transmission of the pain signal. This is the basis of the TENS (transcutaneous electrical nerve stimulation) machines in which electrical stimulation of the skin reduces back pain or labour pain, for example. The pain signal can also be increased or decreased by nerve pathways that originate in the brain and descend down the spinal cord.

So is the transmission and modification of pain signals in the spinal cord abnormal in people with IBS?

A study from France has elegantly demonstrated this. How the spinal cord modifies signals can be seen by studying reflexes, which only need to travel through the spinal cord and are not affected by the brain. One such reflex, called the RIII reflex, involves stimulating a small nerve in the foot with an electric current. The signal from this nerve, travelling up the spinal cord, elicits a small reflex contraction in the biceps muscle of the upper arm. This contraction can be measured with electrodes placed over the muscle, and the strength of the contraction is proportional to the painful electric current stimulus applied to the nerve in the foot.

The researchers measured the intensity of this reflex while at the same time inflating a balloon in the subject's rectum. They found that distending the rectum in volunteers without IBS inhibited this reflex by about 50%. This is to be expected as the pain signal from the rectum will compete with the pain signal from the foot. But when the experiment was repeated in 14 people with IBS, the RIII reflex was not inhibited at all but actually increased by about 30%. This clearly shows an unconscious modification of pain signals in the spinal cord and of an effect in people with IBS that would result in a stronger pain signal reaching the brain.

What happens in the brain?

Our understanding of how signals from the body are processed in the brain has progressed in recent years with the development of 'functional' brain scanning. These scans provide measures of activity in various parts of the brain in response to stimuli applied to other parts of the body.

In positron emission tomography (PET) scanning, for example, slightly radioactive glucose is injected into the bloodstream. As the glucose is used up (metabolised), gamma radiation is emitted and detected by the scanner. The more radiation emitted by an area of brain, the greater the metabolic activity in that area, and metabolic activity is thought to represent nerves that are busy working. In functional magnetic resonance imaging (MRI), blood flow or oxygen use provides a measure of activity. We can combine knowledge gained from these scans with our existing knowledge of the function of different parts of the brain, which has come from anatomical studies and from studies of the results of injury.

Nerve pathways from the body carrying pain signals ascend through the spinal cord to reach various centres in the brain that serve different functions. For example, spatial localisation (identifying which part of the body is sending a signal) is performed by the somatosensory cortex, while pain intensity is defined mainly in an area called the insula, and emotion is added by the anterior cingulate cortex. The signal from these areas is combined and, if strong enough, is consciously perceived.

Are there any differences between pain arising in the gastrointestinal organs and pain arising in the more external parts of the body such as the skin, muscle and bone?

There are two important differences. First, signals from the visceral (internal) organs such as the intestine are very poorly localised. A painful stimulation of a limb will show on a PET scan as an increase in activity in just the part of the somatosensory cortex that deals with that limb. By contrast, painful distension of part of the intestine will lead to a diffuse, more widespread, increase in activity within the somatosensory cortex on both sides of the brain. This is not that surprising as we already know that people can tell very accurately which part of the outside of their body is hurting but find it very difficult to localise pain from their internal organs.

The second difference between gastrointestinal pain and pain from elsewhere in the body is that gastrointestinal pain evokes more intense activity in the anterior cingulate cortex. This is the part of the brain that mediates the emotional element of pain. It is well known that gastrointestinal pain evokes strong emotional responses. It is a more difficult pain to control and is frequently associated with depression. This may be part of the explanation for the difficulty in controlling IBS pain, and the association of IBS with psychological distress.

If IBS is more common in women, does this mean there is a difference in how gastrointestinal sensations are processed in the female brain?

Brain imaging studies have been inconsistent, but it is beginning to look as though women have a greater activation of the anterior cingulate cortex than men in response to gastrointestinal pain. As described in an earlier answer, this is the part of the brain that mediates the emotional element of pain. The implication is that women have an enhanced emotional input to the pain signal.

And are there any differences in how the brain processes gastrointestinal sensations in people with IBS?

Several studies have compared brain activity using PET and functional MRI scans in people with IBS and people without IBS (controls – an earlier answer explains why these are needed). Such studies can be difficult to interpret though. They can involve lying in a noisy claustrophobic MRI scanner waiting for a large balloon that has been inserted into the rectum to be painfully distended. Consequently, they are likely to be affected by the stress this causes in the volunteer. Even so, these studies have tended to show increased activity in the anterior cingulate cortex in people with IBS, implying an increased emotional input to the pain signal.

Interestingly, a recent study of women with IBS has shown that treatment with low-dose amitriptyline reduced activity in the anterior cingulate cortex in response to rectal distension. Amitriptyline is an antidepressant frequently used in low doses to help the pain of IBS.

Can you summarise how visceral hypersensitivity might explain IBS?

The suggestion is that something happens in the intestine – an infection, infestation, inflammation of some sort, an allergic response or even just a change in the normal bacterial flora (the bacteria that live in the gut) following antibiotic use. The chemicals that bring about the inflammation and the hormones secreted as part of the inflammatory response then increase the sensitivity of the sensory mechanisms within the gut. Therefore, the usual functioning of the gut will generate a stronger signal.

Signals from the gut are more capable of initiating an emotional response than signals from other parts of the body. It is reasonable too to suppose that in people who are stressed, anxious or depressed for any reason, this emotional response will be greater. The emotional response integrates with the sensory signal, amplifying it. This amplification can occurs in the brain itself, as well as in the spinal cord, where the nerves are influenced by pathways descending from the brain.

Everyday events within the bowel can now generate sensory signals that, when overamplified, manifest as pain. It is reasonable to suppose that these overamplified signals themselves generate reflex responses that lead to disordered function, diarrhoea, constipation and bloating. The disordered function will generate still stronger sensory signals, which sets up a vicious circle. At times of stress, the symptoms are likely to be worse because the emotional input to the pain signal will be greater. It is also probable that the effects of any food intolerances or allergies will be magnified.

Visceral hypersensitivity, together with the fact that the brain processes signals from the gut in a different manner, is the leading hypothesis in IBS. It covers many of the other theories and features of IBS, and can provide the basis and rationale for further research and treatment.

What are the limitations of visceral hypersensitivity to explain IBS?

There is evidence to back up several aspects of the visceral hypersensitivity story. We know that inflammation can sensitise sensory mechanisms, and we can demonstrate excess sensitivity to distension of the intestine. How closely this mimics IBS is, however, unknown as pain is frequently thought to arise from strong contractions rather than excessive distension.

Furthermore, the concept of hypersensitivity has itself been questioned. When a volunteer in an experiment has a balloon inflated in her rectum, she knows that it might cause pain. If she has IBS, she may have an even greater expectation of pain. The apparent hypersensitivity may thus be just a heightened expectation of pain. This bias can be avoided by doing a large inflation, a small inflation and a sham inflation (no inflation at all) in a random order so the volunteer cannot guess what is coming next. In such experiments, people with

IBS do not feel the balloon at lower volumes than normal, as would be expected from the hypersensitivity theory. Instead, they report any sensation as unpleasant or painful, suggesting that they get pain because they expect it.

It is also unclear just how sensory hypersensitivity results in disordered function. Indeed, there are people with IBS in whom pain is a relatively minor feature compared with the disordered bowel habit or bloating. So why do the symptoms vary so much between different people, and why do they change with time? Finally, why does the hypersensitivity persist? Much remains mysterious.

What are the implications of the 'visceral hypersensitivity' theory for me?

The theory explains how people with symptoms can have completely normal medical tests. This is something that often worries people with IBS. Moreover, it explains how a person's emotional state

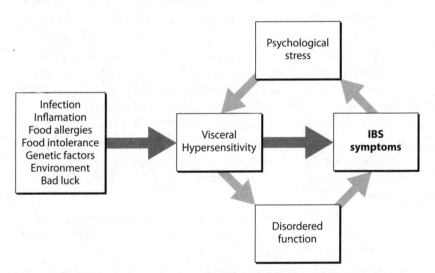

Figure 3.1 The many causes of irritable bowel syndrome.

can affect the severity of the symptoms. Finally, a better understanding of how the gut and the brain interact will allow us to develop new treatments. Some new drugs are already becoming available (see Chapter 4).

Could I have more than one cause for my IBS?

It seems likely that IBS is the culmination of many factors (Figure 3.1). For example, a simple infection may lead to visceral hypersensitivity, exacerbated by stress. Or a mild food intolerance may combine with small bowel bacterial overgrowth to produce profound diarrhoea. A multiplicity of factors combining to cause IBS may explain why there is no simple solution and why the symptoms vary between people and over time.

SUMMARY

- There is a psychological element to IBS in many people. It may not be the cause of the IBS, but it can prolong and exacerbate the symptoms.

- Small bowel bacterial overgrowth – an excess of bacteria in the normally sterile small bowel – may be part of the aetiology of IBS. It should be particularly considered in those with diabetes, people who have had abdominal surgery and the elderly. It may cause diarrhoea-predominant IBS. It is treated by antibiotics.

- Food intolerance or allergy can produce the symptoms of IBS, but whether it causes IBS or is something separate is unknown. A dietary approach will work for some people, some of the time, to a certain extent.

- Subtle inflammation in the bowel wall may be part of the aetiology of IBS, but current anti-inflammatory medication does not work for IBS.

- Visceral hypersensitivity is the concept of enhanced perception, or enhanced responsiveness within the gut – even to everyday events.

- Nerve signals from the gut are more capable of initiating an emotional response than are signals from other parts of the body.

- The emotional response integrates with the sensory signal, amplifying it. This amplification can occur in the brain itself, as well as in the spinal cord, where the nerves are influenced by nerve pathways descending from the brain.

- Our increasing understanding of how the gut and the brain are linked will lead to new treatments in the future.

- IBS may have more than one cause.

4 | Pain in IBS

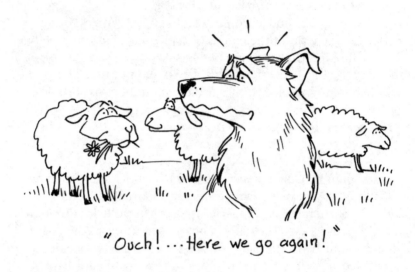

"Ouch! ...Here we go again!"

Pain is essential to our existence. People who lose pain sensation in a limb, because of a nerve injury or a degeneration of their nerves, as can happen in diabetes, can sustain a bad burn or other injury without even realising that anything has happened. Similarly, people can have a completely painless heart attack and be unaware that they have heart disease until their heart finally fails. Pain tells us about injury, and our fear of pain keeps us out of mischief! The paradox of pain is that, at times, it lasts for long after the injury, or occurs without any injury or damage. It then no longer has a useful purpose. Rather than being an important survival mechanism, it becomes a debilitating problem that interferes with our lives.

THE NATURE OF PAIN

I keep hearing the terms 'acute' and 'chronic' pain. What do these mean?

The terms 'acute' and 'chronic' refer to timing rather than severity. 'Acute' implies that the pain is of rapid onset but not prolonged; 'chronic' implies that the pain persists past the usual course of an injury, or recurs every few days weeks or months. The pain of irritable bowel syndrome (IBS) is usually thought of as chronic.

Are there any general differences between acute and chronic pain?

Acute pain is usually caused by some sort of injury such as the trauma of a broken arm, inflammation in an appendix, or the death of a portion of heart muscle, as in a heart attack. Although we expect the severity of the pain to be in proportion to the degree of damage to our body, this isn't always the case. In acute pain, nerve pathways descending from the brain to the spinal cord help to cut down the passage of pain signals to the brain. This is presumably an evolutionary adaptation to allow us to continue to function in the short term despite our injury. In addition, acute pain is often accompanied by a heightened state of awareness and activity.

By contrast, chronic pain may happen without any apparent injury, or even after something has been removed – for example, the 'phantom leg' pain that can occur after amputation. Moreover, it is thought that the descending nerve pathways from the brain no longer help to lessen the pain signal but may instead increase it. Thus, the pain signal that occurs in the spinal cord can be modified so that the nerve cells seem to become hypersensitive. Signals arising from normal function are amplified to the level of pain. In IBS, this phenomenon has come to be known as 'visceral hypersensitivity' (visceral refers to the internal organs, particularly the intestine; see Chapter 3).

Do acute and chronic pain make us behave and feel differently?

A cute pain usually stimulates people into action. Chronic pain is frequently accompanied by lethargy and depression.

Do these two types of pain respond equally well to painkillers?

S adly, chronic pain responds relatively poorly to painkillers (analgesics), but it does better with antidepressants.

Table 4.1 lists the differences between acute and chronic pain.

What are the typical symptoms of IBS pain?

T he symptoms vary widely between people, and even in the same person over time. In order to be able to compare research studies better, conferences of gastroenterologists (doctors specialising in the gut) have been run to agree on diagnostic criteria for IBS. These conferences were held in Rome, and their deliberations are currently known as the 'Rome III criteria' (Box 4.1). The rationale for these criteria is to relate the symptoms to abnormal bowel function. If there aren't any 'alarm symptoms' or abnormalities on physical examination, the diagnosis is almost certainly IBS.

Table 4.1 Differences between acute and chronic pain

Acute pain	Chronic pain
Usually associated with tissue injury	Usually no tissue injury
Heightened state of arousal and activity	Depression and lethargy
Responds well to analgesics	Responds poorly to analgesics
Antidepressants ineffective	Antidepressants can be very effective

Box 4.1 THE DIAGNOSTIC CRITERIA FOR IRRITABLE BOWEL SYNDROME (IBS) BASED ON THE ROME III CONFERENCE (2006)

Recurrent abdominal pain or discomfort for at least 3 days per month in the last 3 months associated with two or more of the following features:

1 Improvement with defecation

2 An onset associated with a change in frequency of the stool

3 An onset associated with a change in form (appearance) of the stool

Other symptoms that together support the diagnosis of IBS include:

- An unusual frequency of the stools (more than three a day, or fewer than three a week)

- An abnormal form of the stools (hard/lumpy or loose/watery; see Figure 7.1 in Chapter 7)

- Abnormal passage of the stools

- The passage of mucus

- Bloating or a feeling of abdominal distension

How do the key symptoms of IBS relate to bowel function?

Table 4.2 gives you information on this.

My doctor said something about the 'right iliac fossa' being a common site for pain in IBS. What is the right iliac fossa?

The right iliac fossa is in the lower right quadrant of the abdomen. There are various systems for describing the location of pain in the abdomen (see Figures 4.1 and 4.2), and most doctors use whichever term seems to describe the pain best. The simplest system involves dividing the abdomen into four quadrants by vertical and

Table 4.2 Interpreting symptoms of irritable bowel syndrome (IBS)

Symptom	Chronic pain
The abdominal pain isn't as bad after defecation	The pain comes from the lower bowel and may be due to distension
The abdominal pain is worse following defecation. (Although this isn't in the Rome III criteria, it is a common symptom)	The pain is from the lower bowel and may be due to spasm
When there are pains, the stools become looser and or more frequent	The functioning of the intestine has altered
Bloating increases through the day but settles at night	The bloating is not due to excess fluid, bowel obstruction or any kind of growth. This is very typical of IBS
There is a feeling of incomplete emptying of the rectum after defecation	The rectum is irritable
Some mucus (slime) may be passed from the rectum	The rectum has been irritated, for example through straining

horizontal lines through the umbilicus (belly button). A more accurate system divides the abdomen into nine regions by two vertical and horizontal lines.

The most commonly used terms include the right and left 'iliac fossa', denoting the lowermost parts of the abdomen, and 'epigastric' denoting the uppermost central part.

Where do people most commonly get pain caused by IBS?

The pain is usually in the abdomen, mostly in the lower right corner, which your doctor will call your 'right iliac fossa'. This is where the caecum – the first part of the large bowel – is found (see Figure 1.1). The small intestine opens into the caecum, and the caecum is frequently distended. This is probably why it is a common

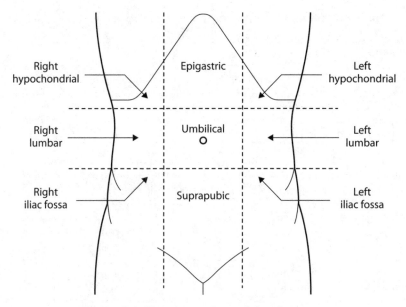

Figure 4.1 The nine regions of the abdomen.

site for pain. Almost as frequent is pain in the left lower corner, the left iliac fossa. This area overlies the sigmoid colon, just above the rectum. It is here that you hold your stool prior to defecation. This area often goes into spasm, and often becomes distended as a result of constipation.

Can IBS cause pain anywhere else?

IBS pain can occur anywhere between the nipples and the thighs, front or back. It can be of a stabbing nature, very brief and lasting for only a few seconds, or it can be spread over a wider area and be poorly localised, which means you can't put your finger on the single spot where the pain is coming from.

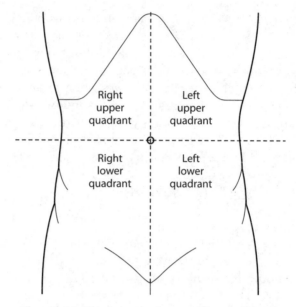

Figure 4.2 The four quadrants of the abdomen.

Is the pain always the same?

No, unlike the pain from diseases with a structural abnormality (cancer, an ulcer, bowel obstruction, etc.), in which the nature, location and character of the pain are always the same, IBS pain can vary in both location and severity.

What's actually causing my pain?

Your pain is probably due to strong contractions of your bowel, or your gut may be distended by faeces or gas. But it may also simply reflect your gut's normal function.

How often do people normally get symptoms from IBS?

There are no hard-and-fast rules. Symptoms may disappear for weeks or months, and then reappear in clusters with a bad week or two. They are often better during times when you can relax, such as holidays, and worse when things are stressful. In one survey of 59 people with IBS over a 12-week period, most reported at least one symptom on over 50% of days, with pain or discomfort on 33% of days, bloating on 28% of days, and altered stool form on 25% of days.

Why is it worse when I'm stressed?

More than any other of our senses, pain is integrated with our emotions. Nerve pathways from centres in the brain that deal with emotion can amplify or reduce the pain signals. This occurs within the brain and also in the spinal cord before the pain signal reaches the brain.

What's the difference between IBS and functional abdominal pain syndrome?

Functional abdominal pain syndrome (also called chronic idiopathic abdominal pain or chronic functional abdominal pain) is fortunately uncommon. It is a severe pain that occurs daily and disrupts normal daily activities. Unlike the pain of IBS, it is not related to bowel function. Moreover, it can last into the night and disturb sleep, something that is unusual for IBS. It is usually associated with psychological problems that are obvious to the doctor but are often minimised or denied by the patient, who is desperate to discover a physical cause for the pain. The cause of this syndrome is unknown.

TREATMENT

Do simple painkillers work for IBS pain?

The simple painkillers (analgesics) that can be purchased at the chemist's do not work for IBS pain. If they *do* work on you, you should question the diagnosis. Codeine-based analgesics (such as codeine phosphate and dihydrocodeine) and paracetamol/codeine combinations (for example, co-codamol, co-dydramol, Kapake, Solpadol and Tylex) are to some extent helpful but usually cause constipation. Codeine-based medicines can be the beginning of a vicious circle, with constipation making the pain worse, so the person takes more tablets, so the constipation gets worse still.

I once had an injection of pethidine and it worked really well for my pain. But my doctor wouldn't give me any more. Why is that?

Pethidine is a potent opiate analgesic. Doctors are extremely reluctant to use opiates in conditions with chronic pain, fearing that physical dependence and addiction may develop. This may seem a little paternalistic and cruel, but all doctors have seen patients who, after receiving ill-advised treatment with an opiate, find themselves having to contend both with the original illness and a drug addiction.

'Opiate' refers to drugs originally produced from the immature seed capsules of the opium poppy plant. Our nervous system produces its own opiate-like chemicals called endorphins. Their principal role is to reduce pain, and many of the cells involved in pain processing have receptors for the endorphin molecules on their surface. These receptors also interact with opiate drugs and have therefore been called 'opiate receptors'. In the bowel, however, activation of these opiate receptors leads to relaxation of the bowel muscle and a profound slowing in function. This is why opiate-based analgesics (painkillers) such as codeine and morphine can cause severe constipation, and why opiate-based drugs can relieve diarrhoea. Codeine is a weak opiate, but pethidine, morphine and diamorphine are all potent opiates. They are very powerful painkillers.

There are several problems with using opiate drugs, including tolerance, physical dependence and addiction. Tolerance means that the body gets used to the drug, so that an increasing dose is required to produce the same effect over time. This doesn't matter if the drug is being given for a short period for acute pain, such as after an operation, or if the patient has a terminal condition. However, it becomes a real problem if the opiate is taken for conditions that last a lifetime.

Physical dependence means that if the drug is stopped suddenly after having been taken long term, usually 1 month or longer, withdrawal symptoms can arise. These include severe anxiety, an unstable mood and physical symptoms such as palpitations, sweating and nausea.

Addiction is a form of psychological dependence – people find that they cannot manage psychologically without the drug and resort to extreme behaviour to get it and take it.

This does not mean that all or even any of these problems will arise in individuals taking opiates for prolonged periods, particularly when they are taken for acute pain. But problems occur often enough for great care to be needed with the use of these drugs.

Smooth muscle relaxants (antispasmodics)

My doctor's said I ought to try a smooth muscle relaxant. What is this?

Smooth muscle relaxants are medicines that are believed to relax the smooth muscle of the bowel, that is, the muscle in the wall of the bowel. They work either directly on the muscle or by inhibiting the nerves that stimulate the gut muscles (in which case they are known as anticholinergic or antimuscarinic drugs). They are believed to reduce the pain of IBS by treating and preventing spasm. Table 4.3 lists some of these.

Table 4.3 Antispasmodic drugs

Drug	Trade names in the UK	Method of action
Dicycloverine (previously called dicyclomine)	Merbentyl Kolanticon gel (this also contains antacids, which neutralise acid in the stomach)	Anticholinergic
Hyoscine	Buscopan	
Propantheline bromide	Pro-Banthine	
Mebeverine	Colofac	Direct smooth muscle relaxation
Alverine citrate	Spasmonal	
Peppermint oil	Colpermin Mintec	

Do these smooth muscle relaxants have any side effects?

They are believed to be safe and mostly free of side effects. Most are available without prescription. Anticholinergic drugs can cause a dry mouth, blurred vision and constipation if they are used in higher doses. Anticholinergic drugs should not be used by people with glaucoma (increased pressure within the eyes), and they can occasionally cause elderly people to become confused. In the doses used for IBS, however, there are usually no significant side effects. Peppermint oil can sometimes cause heartburn.

But do they work?

Yes, in some people, some of the time and to some extent. There have been many studies of these preparations in people with IBS. The studies are, however, difficult to interpret because the 'placebo response rate' – the number of people who improve while taking the sham drug (see Chapter 12) – in IBS trials varies from 20% to over 80%. But in most trials, the muscle relaxant was better than the placebo, and so it's definitely worth trying them as they may help to relieve your symptoms.

When should I take my antispasmodics?

You should take them about 30 minutes before meals as they take that length of time to work. You can take them regularly or intermittently. They combine well with other medications and treatments for IBS. Try different antispasmodics to find one that works for you.

Antidepressants

Low-dose tricyclic antidepressants

These are possibly the most potent medicines for IBS pain.

What are tricyclic antidepressants?

These were the first group of antidepressant drugs that really worked and were relatively safe. Amitriptyline was the first of the group and has been in use for over 50 years. Exactly how they work is still unclear, but they seem to increase the levels of the transmitters noradrenaline (norepinephrine) and serotonin within the brain by preventing them being taken up again by cells once they have been secreted. This gives them longer to act.

Are they analgesics?

You would not take tricyclic antidepressants for a twisted ankle, so they are not analgesic in the sense that they reduce acute pain. But they do reduce chronic pain and are extremely useful for this.

Early on in the history of these drugs, it was noticed that some people with depression felt less pain soon after starting a tricyclic, long before their depression lifted. There is now compelling evidence that the activity of these medicines against chronic pain is independent of their effect on depression and occurs at much lower doses. Tricyclics take 2–3 weeks or more to lift a depression, but may work for pain almost immediately. Some individuals notice a benefit within a day, although 3–7 days is more common.

I'm not sure what dose of amitriptyline I should be taking. What is meant by a low dose?

The starting dose of amitriptyline for depression is 75 mg (milligrams). This dose can be gradually increased in depression to 200 mg each day. By contrast, the starting dose for pain and IBS is usually 10 mg a day. This dose is often successful, but if not, it can be increased by 10–25 mg every week. For IBS, I usually recommend a maximum of 50 mg a day, although it has been used for pain in higher doses.

Is low-dose amitriptyline used to treat any other pains?

It is used for most conditions in which chronic pain is a problem, including rheumatoid arthritis, back pain, sciatica, headaches and cancer-related pain.

Does it have to be taken all the time?

It has to be taken continuously for depression and should not be stopped suddenly. But this is not the case when it is used for pain. It may work better if it is taken continuously, but it can be used intermittently. Many people taking low-dose amitriptyline stop and restart it depending on what sort of a week they are having. If you are taking more than a very low dose, for instance more than 50 mg a day, you would probably be better off tapering the dose down over a week rather than stopping it suddenly. The pain does not rebound (bounce back worse) if it is stopped.

I'm worried that I could get addicted to my tricyclics.
Could that happen?

No, they're not addictive. There are people whose depression rebounds if they stop taking the drug, but otherwise there are usually no withdrawal effects. Most family doctors will have a lot of experience in using these types of medication. You should not hesitate to seek their advice.

What are the side effects?

Side effects are unfortunately common with tricyclic antidepressants. They usually cause drowsiness, a dry mouth, blurred vision, constipation, urinary retention (difficulty passing urine) and sexual dysfunction. The drowsiness may be apparent even with the very low doses used for pain in IBS. It may be better to take them at night, but you should start the medication at a weekend as the drowsiness can last into the next day. Tricyclics usually help you to sleep, but occasionally they disturb sleep, sometimes causing nightmares. When the tablets are taken continuously, however, the side effects wear off after 2–3 weeks. In the long term, some people complain of weight gain.

In larger doses, tricyclics can cause serious side effects with abnormal heart rhythms in people with heart disease or more convulsions in people with epilepsy. They are dangerous in overdose because of their effect on the heart.

I tend to be very susceptible to side effects from drugs; I doubt
if I would tolerate amitriptyline.

It's interesting that some people with IBS are intolerant of many drugs because of side effects. However, if you have a lot of trouble with IBS, it's much better for you to try amitriptyline than avoid it. The smallest size tablet is 10 mg, and you can also get it as a syrup (25 mg in each 5 ml spoonful). Start with 10 mg at night, or less if you can break the tablet. This is a very small dose compared with what is prescribed for depression (75–150 mg a day), and most people will have minimal side effects. If you take it continuously and try to work through any side effects, the side effects will wear off, but your IBS will continue to improve.

I'm finding it really hard to cope with the drowsiness that my amitriptyline causes. Are the other tricyclic antidepressants any better?

In short, yes. Amitriptyline has been the best studied with respect to pain management, but the other tricyclics probably work just as well. Amoxapine, imipramine, lofepramine and nortriptyline are all less sedative than amitriptyline, which means that they cause less drowsiness. Lofepramine also causes less of a dry mouth. The starting dose of lofepramine for depression is 140 mg, and it is only available as 70 mg tablets or as a syrup containing 70 mg in each 5 ml spoonful, so start with 35 mg a day. Imipramine (similar to desipramine (US)) is dosed in the same levels as amitriptyline and is available in 10 mg tablets.

Would a full dose of a tricyclic antidepressant work better for IBS than a low dose?

It may be worthwhile slowly increasing the dose to the full antidepressant dose. For instance, the doctor can increase your dose of amitriptyline by 10–25 mg every week or so up to 150 mg a day for a normal adult. The problem is that, at that dose, it will cause constipation. This may be to your advantage if your problem is diarrhoea, but otherwise the tricyclic may make your IBS worse.

What antidepressant should I use if I'm depressed and constipated?

There's a class of antidepressants called SSRIs (selective serotonin reuptake inhibitors), which rarely cause constipation and are more likely to cause diarrhoea.

Selective serotonin reuptake inhibitors (SSRIs)

What are SSRIs?

Some of the nerve cells in the brain release a transmitter called serotonin (also known as 5-hydroxytryptamine or 5-HT). The SSRIs – citalopram, escitalopram, fluoxetine, fluvoxamine, paroxetine and sertraline – selectively stop this serotonin being taken back up again after it has been secreted from the nerves. They therefore increase the levels of serotonin in the brain, and this is thought to be how they work in depression. They are as effective as the tricyclic drugs for depression but usually have far fewer, if any, side effects.

Do SSRIs have an effect on the gut too?

The enteric nervous system (the nervous system of the gut) uses much more serotonin than the brain so one would expect SSRIS to have a profound effect on the gut. Surprisingly, however, although a few patients have some gastrointestinal side effects such as diarrhoea, nausea and lack of appetite, most people notice little if any change in their gut function.

Could SSRIs help my IBS?

SSRIs are very helpful in people with IBS who are also depressed, and they are then used continuously in full doses. But for pain they are probably less effective than low-dose tricyclics.

Could I take SSRIs and tricyclics together?

Doctors do occasionally use a full dose of an SSRI for depression together with a low dose of a tricyclic for pain. So you may be given both by your doctor, depending on your circumstances, and this may work well for you.

New medicines for IBS

One of the 'problems' in introducing new drugs for IBS is that no one dies from IBS! This may seem a preposterous statement to make, but it does mean that new drugs specifically for IBS have to be virtually 100% safe to be worth taking, and this is probably impossible. New drugs usually act to change the levels of neurotransmitters (transmitters between nerve cells) such as serotonin, which are found throughout the body, being used for different things in different places. So taking a drug that has effects all through the body can cause unexpected consequences.

The problem of introducing new drugs is shown by the case of the drug alosetron (see below). This was withdrawn after a small significant risk of serious, even life-threatening side effects was found, although it was reintroduced after pressure from patient groups and manufacturers. It is not, however, available in the UK.

Alosetron

Alosetron (brand name Lotronex) is a 'selective serotonin 5-HT$_3$ receptor antagonist'. That means that it blocks the action of serotonin on one of its receptors, called the 5-HT$_3$ receptor. The most important action of 5-HT$_3$ receptors is to transmit pain signals from the bowel to the brain by activating sensory nerve cells that are involved in pain sensation in the gut. Serotonin released from other cells in the gut (called enterochromaffin or EC cells) can also stimulate 5-HT$_3$ receptors on an important nerve called the vagus nerve. This can then lead to nausea and non-painful gut sensations, such as bloating and fullness.

Blocking the 5-HT$_3$ receptors may therefore reduce the pain, the need to go to the toilet quickly once you feel you need to (called urgency) and other symptoms associated with the hypersensitivity of diarrhoea-predominant IBS (IBS-D). It can, however, only be used in IBS-D, because it causes constipation.

How effective is alosetron?

There have been a number of clinical trials with alosetron. For example, after 12 weeks of treatment in one of these studies, 76% of people treated with alosetron had a moderate or substantial improvement in their IBS-D symptoms compared with 44% of those treated with a placebo (a sham treatment). This has led some people to claim that alosetron is 'highly efficacious' or even a 'miracle' treatment. Others, however, point out that the number of people responding to the drug in most studies was only 10–20% more than the number who responded to the placebo.

What side effects does alosetron have?

In studies, some side effects occurred more frequently with alosetron than with the placebo treatment. These included constipation (29% versus 6% with placebo), abdominal discomfort or pain (7% versus 4%) and nausea (6% versus 5%). For most people, the constipation was mild and transient, occurred just once during the first month of treatment, and resolved on its own or with a break in treatment.

However, serious side effects also occurred. These included severe complications of constipation, ischaemic colitis, hospitalisation, surgery and death. Complications of constipation occur when faeces are impacted so hard within the bowel that the wall perforates, leading to potentially fatal infections in the body cavity. Ischaemic colitis is the interruption of blood flow to the bowel and can resolve itself without problems or can lead to death of part of the gut and life-threatening complications.

Serious complications related to constipation (e.g. obstruction, perforation, impaction or death) occurred in approximately 1 out of every 1000 people taking alosetron. In one study, the risk of ischaemic colitis in women taking it was about 3 in every 1000 women over 6 months. As a result, the manufacturer, GlaxoSmith-Kline, voluntarily withdrew alosetron from the US market in November 2000.

In November 2002, however, alosetron was reintroduced under a restricted-access programme for women with severe IBS-D lasting 6 months or longer who did not have any anatomical or biochemical abnormalities of their gastrointestinal tract and who had failed to respond to traditional therapy. Severe IBS-D, as defined in the package information for alosetron, refers to diarrhoea with one or more of the following features: frequent and severe abdominal pain or discomfort, frequent urgency of stool and incontinence of stool, and disability or restriction of daily activities.

Alosetron is not available in the UK.

Do you think alosetron should be available in the UK?

Nothing is completely safe, and the risks of new drugs are difficult to quantify. If people with severe IBS-D are willing to take what is likely to be a small risk, I believe that this drug should be available for them to try.

Tegaserod maleate

What is tegaserod?

Tegaserod (brand name Zelnorm) is a 'selective serotonin type 4 ($5-HT_4$) receptor partial agonist'. That's a bit of a mouthful but just means that it partially mimics the action of serotonin at one of its receptors. This receptor can be found on the muscle cells of the gut and on nerve cells that supply the gut. When it is activated, it stimulates peristalsis (co-ordinated contractions of the muscles of the gut to propel the contents along) and the secretion of water and digestive juices into the gut. It is therefore used for women with IBS whose primary bowel symptom is constipation (IBS-C). Activation of the $5-HT_4$ receptor may also reverse visceral hypersensitivity (see earlier in the chapter, and also Chapter 3) and reduce pain.

Tegaserod is not yet licensed for treatment in the UK.

How effective is tegaserod?

In clinical trials involving mainly women with IBS-C, up to 50% had either considerable or complete relief of their constipation, and about 40% had relief from pain. Most of the benefit occurred within a few weeks of starting treatment. The placebo effect (the improvement occurring through the use of sham medication) was, however, also high. In three trials including a total of 2470 women, about 14% more women benefited from tegaserod compared with the placebo after 1 month of treatment.

Statistically, these results were highly significant, so it seems likely that tegaserod will be successful in a proportion of people with severe constipation. Those with severe IBS-C who do not respond to current medical treatment are often desperate to find something that will help them put their life back on track, so it's frustrating that tegaserod is not yet licensed in the UK.

Can men use tegaserod too?

They probably can, but it has been mainly tested on women. It is not yet apparent whether this will have any implications when tegaserod is finally licensed.

What are the side effects of tegaserod?

Mild diarrhoea especially in the first week of treatment was the most frequent adverse event: it affected 9–33% of people who took tegaserod. Other reported adverse events included abdominal pain, nausea and headache. These side effects occurred just as often with tegaserod as with placebo so may reflect the IBS more than the treatment.

There have been isolated reports of ischaemic colitis in patients taking tegaserod. Ischaemic colitis is a serious inflammation of the wall of the large bowel that occurs when there is not enough blood supply. It is an uncommon condition even in people with a poor circulation, and may possibly occur as a consequence of longstanding severe constipation. It is not yet clear whether the reports of ischaemic colitis in people taking tegaserod are a coincidence and nothing to do with the drug, or whether ischaemic colitis is a real risk with tegaserod. In any case, the risk is likely to be very small.

Do you think tegaserod should be available in the UK?

As I said in an earlier answer, nothing is completely safe, and the risks of new drugs are difficult to assess. If people with severe IBS-C are willing to take what is probably a small risk, I believe that this drug should be made available for them to try.

Melatonin

What is melatonin?

Melatonin is closely related to serotonin (5-HT; see earlier in the chapter). It is secreted by the pineal gland in the brain and may have a function in controlling the sleep–wake cycle. Its secretion is enhanced during darkness and suppressed during daylight. Melatonin has been found to have a sleep-promoting effect and is promoted as being helpful for jet lag.

Is melatonin useful for IBS?

Only one small study from Singapore has tested melatonin on people with IBS who also had disturbed sleep. A dose of 3 mg of melatonin was used each night for 2 weeks and then compared with a placebo (sham treatment). Interestingly, the melatonin failed to improve sleep. However, there was a significant improvement in abdominal pain and rectal sensitivity. Stool frequency, stool form and bloating were not improved.

Can I get melatonin easily?

Melatonin is *not* an established treatment for IBS. I have mentioned it here because melatonin is available in most countries, like the UK, without prescription and is regarded as safe.

Are any other drugs being developed?

There are several drugs in the early stages of development and testing.

Cilansetron is a new 'selective serotonin 5-HT$_3$ receptor antagonist', similar to alosetron (see an earlier question), that is currently being developed. Two trials so far have shown it to be beneficial in IBS-D. However, the UK's Medicines and Healthcare products Regulatory Agency and the US Food and Drug Administration have asked for further trials before they will approve it.

Renazapride is a new drug being developed for all types of IBS. It has a serotonin 5-HT$_4$ receptor agonist effect similar to that of tegaserod, as well as a 5-HT$_3$ receptor antagonist action. It may combine the beneficial actions of both the new drugs discussed above, similar to alosetron. A study involving 1700 women with IBS-C is currently being planned in the USA.

Asimadoline is a drug called a kappa opioid that may help with symptoms of pain. Unlike other opioid drugs such as morphine or codeine, asimadoline only works on one of the three opioid receptors. The kappa receptor only exists outside the brain, and asimadoline does not cross into the brain, so it doesn't have a sedative effect and shouldn't be addictive.

Talnetant is called a neurokinin-3 antagonist. It may help with the oversensitivity of the muscles in the colon.

CONCLUSION

Pain is not always present in IBS, and in some people it is not a major factor. In others, it can be severe and impossible to ignore. It can also be difficult to accept that severe pain is not a consequence of a serious problem – it's all to easy to think that the pain of IBS must be due to a 'blockage' or 'a growth'. It is all the more worrying as simple analgesics (painkillers) fail to work here.

Visceral hypersensitivity, or how the normal function of internal organs can manifest as pain, is discussed in Chapter 3 on the causes of IBS. Pain in IBS does not represent physical damage. But it is not a purely psychological phenomenon either. It may be thought of as a 'signalling problem' between the gut and the brain. As a result, simple analgesics do not work. Smooth muscle relaxant drugs, called antispasmodics (see earlier in the chapter), work to some extent by reducing spasm and dampening down strong contractions. Codeine and other opiate-based drugs do reduce the pain but at the cost of reducing the gut's muscular activity and propulsion. The resulting constipation will cause worsening pain.

The best treatments for IBS pain modify the signalling pathway between the gut and the brain. Most successful in this respect is treatment with low-dose tricyclic antidepressants. The SSRIs are also worth trying. With our increasing understanding of the signalling pathways, and especially of the role of serotonin, new drugs are becoming available. In the meantime, it is unfortunate but inevitable that people with IBS may have to put up with a degree of chronic pain.

People with IBS should overcome their reluctance to try low-dose amitriptyline and other antidepressants. Most doctors know of individuals whose pain improved dramatically with these medications even after nothing else had worked.

How can my doctor be so sure that my pain is 'nothing to worry about'?

Different diseases present with different symptom patterns. Although there is often an overlap in the symptoms of different illnesses, we can recognise distinct patterns. As the doctor listens to your symptoms, he or she will be looking for distinct patterns that fit particular diseases. There is no mystery to this. The next chapter, on recognising abdominal pain that is not the result of IBS, gives brief descriptions of conditions that cause abdominal pain. Although it isn't comprehensive, it will help you to understand how doctors differentiate the different causes of abdominal pain.

Your doctor will also be listening out for symptoms that suggest more serious pathology, so-called 'alarm symptoms'.

What do doctors mean by 'alarm symptoms'?

These are the symptoms and signs that suggest more serious diseases such as bowel cancer, colitis, Crohn's disease or coeliac disease (Table 4.4). These symptoms call for medical tests. If you have such symptoms, you should see your doctor. The most likely diagnosis may still be IBS simply because it is so common (IBS affects 10–20% of people, whereas the lifetime risk of bowel cancer is only 4%, or 1 in 25 people). Even so, because bowel cancer is one of the more treatable cancers, any change in bowel habit in a person over the age of 50 is investigated.

I've had severe pain for years. The doctors have been useless. All they say is that they can't find anything wrong. I've tried everything going and nothing helps. How can I be expected to live like this?

As you have had the pain for years and the doctors still can't find anything wrong, this means that your pain is 'functional' – it arises out of normal function and does not signify any damage.

Table 4.4 Alarm symptoms suggesting that the diagnosis may not be irritable bowel syndrome (IBS)

Symptom	Comment
Rectal bleeding	Bright red blood suggests that the bleeding is from the lower part of the bowel on the left side of the abdomen
	Blood only on the outside of the stool is likely to be from the rectum
	Blood mixed in with the stool has come from higher up in the bowel
	Darker blood is blood that is partially digested so must be coming from higher up in the bowel
	Shiny, loose, tarry black stools are called 'melaena'. This is blood digested by acid and intestinal juices, and is most likely to have come from the stomach or duodenum
	Although benign conditions such as piles probably account for 90% of bright red rectal bleeding, people who get this symptom should see their doctor to exclude more serious problems
Weight loss	Occasionally, people with IBS lose weight because they eat less to avoid symptoms induced by their meals. Weight loss is also a common feature of depression
Continuous diarrhoea	Diarrhoea can be caused by a huge range of problems, and it is often worthwhile investigating this
Anaemia	This is definitely not a feature of IBS
Recurrent vomiting	This is more likely to be due to a structural stomach problem
Fever	Fever suggests inflammation or infection

Table 4.4 Alarm symptoms suggesting that the diagnosis may not be irritable bowel syndrome (IBS) *continued*

Symptom	Comment
Night-time symptoms, disturbing sleep or waking the person from sleep	These are unusual in IBS
A family history of bowel cancer, Crohn's disease, ulcerative colitis or coeliac disease	One first-degree relative (parent, brother or sister) with bowel cancer doubles your risk of developing it too
	Having a first-degree relative with inflammatory bowel disease or coeliac disease gives you about a 10% risk of getting that disorder
Recent travel to areas with widespread infective gut disease or recent travel	Infection with an organism called *Giardia* is fairly common, and the symptoms are frequently prolonged

Consequently, tests looking for damage from inflammation, cancer, infection, etc. will always be negative.

Because you have lived with this for years, you will probably go on living with it for years. If you have really tried 'everything going' and no doctor or alternative practitioner has helped you, maybe you should work towards accepting your symptoms rather than pursuing a fruitless search for a cure. Save your energy for those parts of your life that are going well. There are many people with ongoing symptoms and disabilities of one sort or another that medicine – conventional or complementary – cannot significantly help. No one has died of IBS, and life **does** go on.

But there must be something else to try?

You're probably right! When people say they have tried everything, it is often more a statement of their frustration than of their actual experience. It is worth making a list of what you have tried, for how long, at what dose and in what circumstances. It may be worth trying some of these treatments again, perhaps in combination. An experienced doctor will probably have several suggestions to make based on your previous experience and your current symptoms. Moreover, new drugs and techniques to deal with IBS will hopefully be increasingly available in the coming years.

SUMMARY

- Acute and chronic pain are different.

- The pain of IBS is usually associated with a change in bowel habit.

- The pain of IBS does not represent physical damage. It should be thought of as a signalling problem between the gut and the brain.

- In IBS there should be no 'alarm' symptoms (e.g. bleeding, anaemia, weight loss or night-time symptoms).

- Simple analgesics like paracetamol or ibuprofen do not usually work in IBS.

- Antispasmodics or smooth muscle relaxants can work, and usually without side effects.

- Low-dose amitriptyline is probably the most effective drug currently available for pain in IBS.

- New drugs are being developed, but their availability is still restricted because of worries about serious side effects.

5 | Recognising abdominal pain that is not due to IBS

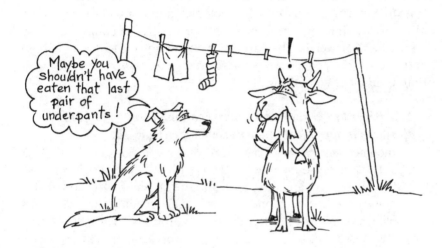

One of the most frequent worries for anyone with irritable bowel syndrome (IBS) is whether there could be anything else wrong. Could it be an ulcer, a cancer, a gall stone? Could I have another condition as well as IBS? Is my IBS 'masking' the symptoms of another condition?

These concerns are entirely understandable, and they are made worse by the fact that there is no specific test for IBS. We diagnose IBS by recognising a conglomeration of symptoms and by performing a limited number of tests to rule out other conditions. It's never possible to completely rule out all possible conditions, so there will always be an element of doubt and uncertainty. There will always be symptoms that are not completely explained, and the question of what else could be going on is often still at the back of people's minds. It may seem to be an impossible situation; no one can have all the tests every time they get somewhat different symptoms.

But in fact most abdominal conditions are recognised by the way people describe their symptoms. The physical examination and the tests are there largely to confirm the diagnosis. Doctors listen out for patterns of symptoms that suggest certain conditions and perform tests to confirm or deny their suspicions. There is no mystery to this. Most of the time, common problems present with common, easily recognisable patterns. The purpose of this chapter is to describe these patterns so that people can begin to answer for themselves the question 'Could it be something else?'

Whenever I read about a disease, I can make my symptoms fit the description. I just make myself more worried.

Yes, that was also me as a medical student! It is the risk you take when you try to find out more. You may wish to write down your symptoms or to keep a symptom diary before reading the rest of this chapter. Or you could describe your symptoms to another, more objective person. Finally, remember that you are not alone; it's very human to worry, and most worries turn out to be unfounded.

When I finally saw my doctor, I found it very difficult to give a coherent description of my pain. I'm afraid he thought me a bit of a fool.

It is not unusual for people to find it difficult to describe their symptoms. It's partly a matter of nerves, and partly not knowing what is and isn't relevant. Doctors expect this and make allowances. Surprisingly, if you have had symptoms for a long time, it can be even more difficult to describe them. We describe what is abnormal for us by contrasting it with what is normal for us; for some people, the symptoms of IBS can become such a part of their normal life that it can be confusing to distinguish the 'normal' from the 'abnormal'.

What do doctors need to know about the nature of the pain in order to make a diagnosis?

Think about your pain before seeing the doctor and prepare answers to these questions:

- How long have you been unwell?

- Where do you get the pain?

- Does it go anywhere else?

- Is it always the same pain, or are there several pains?

- When you get the pain, is it constant or does it come and go in severity?

- How long does it last?

- What makes it better or worse?

- How often do you get it?

- Are you well between episodes of pain?

- Are there any associated symptoms such as nausea, vomiting, diarrhoea, constipation, weight loss or bleeding?

- Have you had anything like this before? What tests and treatment did you have?

- Describe your diet.

- Is there any family history of bowel problems?

- What medications are you taking now? (it's a good idea to take a list with you)

- What medications, prescribed or from the chemist, have you tried? (again, take a list)

GALL STONES

Gall stones floating in the gallbladder usually cause no symptoms. If a gall stone becomes stuck in the duct leading out of the gall bladder (the cystic duct; Figure 5.1), the resulting pain is called biliary colic. If stones within the gall bladder cause inflammation and infection, we get cholecystitis. If a stone passes through the cystic duct but gets stuck in the common bile duct, there is usually no pain, but because the bile cannot flow out to the intestine, the person becomes jaundiced.

Biliary colic

The pain begins unexpectedly in the upper middle abdomen. Because eating causes the gall bladder to contract, the pain may occur after a meal, but it can occur at any time and may wake people from their sleep. The pain builds up over 15 minutes to an hour and can become very severe. It is called a colic, which implies that it comes in waves. But biliary colic is actually almost always a continuous pain. It is very much centred in the upper abdomen, but the pain can spread to the right upper corner of the abdomen and to the back. There is no inflammation so movement does not make the pain worse. Indeed, people often try to move about in the hope of shifting the pain, usually to no avail.

Nausea and vomiting are frequently associated with biliary colic, and this, along with the position of the pain, leads people to think that there might be something seriously amiss with their stomach. The pain is sometimes so high in the abdomen that they wonder whether they are having a heart attack. The pain continues until the stone either disengages or passes through the cystic duct, usually in half an hour to several hours. Although people usually feel rather 'winded' for a few hours after an attack, they are back to normal by the following day.

Attacks of pain only occur if a stone is blocking the cystic duct. This may happen every few weeks or months, but importantly the

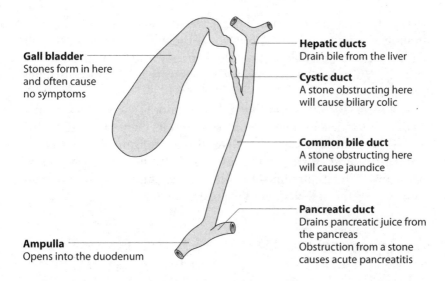

Gall bladder
Stones form in here
and often cause
no symptoms

Hepatic ducts
Drain bile from the liver

Cystic duct
A stone obstructing here
will cause biliary colic

Common bile duct
A stone obstructing here
will cause jaundice

Pancreatic duct
Drains pancreatic juice from
the pancreas
Obstruction from a stone
causes acute pancreatitis

Ampulla
Opens into the duodenum

Figure 5.1 The biliary system. Stones commonly form in the gall bladder.
They can obstruct the cystic duct, causing biliary colic, or pass through
into the common bile duct. Stones can also form or enlarge in the
common bile duct.

stones are just floating in the gall bladder between attacks and there
are no symptoms. This episodic (on-and-off) pattern of biliary colic
contrasts with the symptoms of IBS or indigestion, which tend to
occur to some degree on most days.

The diagnosis of biliary colic is based on typical symptoms plus an
abdominal ultrasound scan demonstrating stones in the gallbladder.
The treatment is surgery to remove the gall bladder (cholecystectomy).

Cholecystitis

If the cystic duct is obstructed for a long time or the gall bladder wall
is irritated by gallstones, the wall of the gall bladder will become
inflamed. The pain is in the right upper corner of the abdomen, and
that site will be very tender if someone presses it. The pain can be

severe and may be, because there is inflammation, made worse by moving or deep breathing. Moreover, if the inflammation of the gall bladder irritates the diaphragm, the pain may also be felt in the right shoulder. There is often a fever, and people with cholecystitis usually look and feel unwell.

In contrast to biliary colic, which lasts for only a few hours, cholecystitis continues for days. It may settle on its own, but it may also require hospital admission. The diagnosis is confirmed by an abdominal ultrasound scan that shows gall stones in a thickened gallbladder. The treatment is to allow the inflammation to settle and then remove the gall bladder by an operation (cholecystectomy).

PANCREATITIS

Pancreatitis is an inflammation of the pancreas most frequently caused by drinking too much alcohol over a period of several years; less often, it is caused by gall stones. Acute pancreatitis occurs suddenly and lasts for a short period of time, usually resolving. Chronic pancreatitis does not improve but results in a slow destruction of the pancreas. Either form can cause serious complications that may be life-threatening.

Acute pancreatitis

The typical attack of acute pancreatitis begins with severe and persistent pain in the upper abdomen that often radiates (spreads) through to the back. It may follow a large meal and is associated with nausea, and persistent vomiting and retching. The pain is worse with movement, so people with it tend to lie still. It is not the sort of pain that allows people to carry on any sort of normal activity, and hospital admission is usually necessary. A simple blood test showing elevated levels of amylase, an enzyme released from the pancreas, confirms the diagnosis. Treatment usually involves intravenous fluids and pain relief for about a week.

Chronic pancreatitis

The pain of chronic pancreatitis may be identical to that of acute pancreatitis, but it may be continuous, intermittent or even absent. Although the classic description is of upper abdominal pain spreading through to the back, a different pattern is often seen: the pain may be worst in the right or left upper corner of the back, it may be spread throughout the upper abdomen, and it may even be felt in the front of the chest or on the person's side. Characteristically, the pain is persistent and deep-seated, and does not respond to antacids. It can be made worse by alcohol or a heavy meal (especially one rich in fat). Often, the pain is severe enough to need frequent, powerful analgesics (painkillers).

The pancreas normally produces digestive juices, and chronic pancreatitis causes a gradual destruction of the pancreas. Consequently, in chronic pancreatitis there is often a failure to digest food properly, especially fat. This results in diarrhoea with loose, pale, offensive-smelling stools and weight loss. In the early stages of the disease, however, there may be a lot of pain but no other symptoms or signs. Diagnosis can therefore be difficult. In contrast to acute pancreatitis, blood tests are usually negative. Ultrasound or CT (computed tomography) scans of the abdomen may also be normal, and more sophisticated tests to show the ducts within the pancreas (called MRCP or ERCP tests) are usually necessary.

Chronic pancreatitis has been mistaken for IBS. This is understandable as both cause persisting abdominal pain and diarrhoea, often on a daily basis. But there are a number of differences that help to distinguish the two conditions (Table 5.1).

STOMACH AND DUODENAL ULCERS

The pain is in the upper abdomen. It is usually described as a sharp or burning pain that is disturbing but not severe enough to incapacitate someone in the way that biliary colic or pancreatitis might. It

Table 5.1 Some clinical differences between irritable bowel syndrome and chronic pancreatitis

	Irritable bowel syndrome	Chronic pancreatitis
Pain at night	Unusual	Common
Diarrhoea at night	Very unusual	Common
Weight loss	Very unusual	Common
Current or previous alcohol abuse	Unusual	75% of patients
Pale, fatty, offensive-smelling diarrhoea	Unusual	Common
Diarrhoea responds to one or two capsules of loperamide	Common	Unusual
Diarrhoea responds to pancreatic enzyme supplements	Unusual	Common

used to be thought that duodenal and gastric ulcers could be distinguished by the timing of the pain in relation to food, duodenal ulcers being characterised by pain when the person was starving hungry, and relieved by meals, gastric ulcer pain being brought on by food, so that people avoided meals and lost weight. There is some truth in this, but the symptoms are often not as clear cut.

When all the many symptoms attributed to duodenal ulcers are carefully analysed, the one that discriminates best (although by no means 100%) is upper abdominal pain that wakes the person in the middle of the night and is relieved by taking antacids or milk. With gastric ulcers, the symptoms occur sooner after food, and vomiting and weight loss are more common, whereas they are rare with an uncomplicated duodenal ulcer.

Ulcers occur in the stomach and duodenum because of the acidic environment. Reducing the acidity with medication quickly abolishes the pain and allows the ulcer to heal. Traditional antacids that neutralise some of the acid in the stomach are only mildly effective. Drugs that reduce acid secretion into the stomach, such as omeprazole or ranitidine, are dramatically effective at reducing and then abolishing the pain within a few days. If these drugs have no effect, the pain is very unlikely to be due to an ulcer.

GASTRO-OESOPHAGEAL REFLUX (ACID REFLUX)

In this condition, acid from the stomach flows back (refluxes up) into the oesophagus. A hiatus hernia (a bulging of the stomach up through the diaphragm and into the chest) allows this to happen more easily, but acid reflux is very common and happens even with completely normal anatomy. Acid in the oesophagus causes a painful or burning sensation in the upper abdomen or chest, often described as heartburn (Figure 5.2). It can occasionally be felt in the back, but

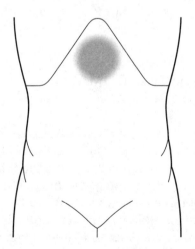

Figure 5.2 Epigastric pain. Pain at this site can occur in a number of conditions, including gastric and duodenal ulcers, gastro-oesophageal reflux, dysmotility of the stomach, biliary colic and irritable bowel syndrome.

at other times there is no chest pain and it becomes difficult to distinguish it from ulcer pain. Sometimes the pain is only in the chest and can be severe enough to suggest a heart attack.

Symptoms typically occur after eating a large or fatty meal or drinking alcohol or coffee. Lying down, bending over or bending and lifting can all make it worse. Smoking, being overweight and pregnancy all contribute to reflux, but it can occur without any obvious cause and is the most common cause of indigestion. The frequency of symptoms varies. For most people, symptoms occur only occasionally, but there can be weekly or daily episodes of reflux. A gastroscope examination, in which a doctor puts a tube with a miniature camera on it down the person's oesophagus, may show inflammation in the oesophagus from acid reflux, but in at least a third of cases the oesophagus and stomach look entirely normal.

As with ulcers, treatment with drugs that reduce acid secretion into the stomach, such as omeprazole or ranitidine, is dramatically effective at reducing and then abolishing the pain, usually within a few days. If these drugs have no effect, the pain is very unlikely to be due to acid reflux.

DYSMOTILITY OF THE STOMACH (NON-ULCER DYSPEPSIA)

The term 'non-ulcer dyspepsia' refers to indigestion symptoms in people who do not have simple reflux, ulcers, inflammation or structural problems in their oesophagus or stomach. It is thought to be mainly due to poor co-ordination of the muscles in the stomach (dysmotility) and responds only partly or not at all to drugs that reduce acid secretion. It is not IBS, which is a mainly disorder of the large bowel, but can be thought of as an IBS-type syndrome affecting the upper gastrointestinal tract.

Dysmotility (meaning bad movement) of the stomach is actually a very common disorder that few people have heard about. Poor co-ordination of the muscles in the stomach results in a variety of symptoms that can be misinterpreted as an irritable bowel. Mechanically, the stomach works as two parts. The upper part dilates to hold food coming down from the oesophagus. The lower part is controlled by a pacemaker that sends electric signals to the muscle, causing it to contract rhythmically and churn the food.

But both parts may fail to function normally. If the upper part fails to dilate to make enough room for the food, we feel full early on in the meal ('early satiety'). Continuing to eat causes a feeling of pressure in the upper abdomen, which some people describe as bloating. There may also be some reflux of acid or food.

The lower part of the stomach may fail in several ways. The electrical signal from the pacemaker may temporarily stop altogether. It feels as though the food is just sitting in the stomach, and there may be upper abdominal bloating and nausea. We sometimes call this prolonged digestion, but it may feel worse than that name suggests. The electrical signal from the stomach pacemaker may also be too active. In this case, the stomach contractions may be too vigorous, causing pain, nausea and excess noise.

There is no specific test for dysmotility. Gastroscope examinations of the stomach and blood tests are normal. In retrospect, people usually realise that they have had the symptoms for a long time, but there is no weight loss and physical examination is normal. The combination of early satiety, bloating, prolonged digestion and often nausea and reflux strongly suggests the diagnosis.

Drugs that reduce acid secretion may be partly helpful but are frequently disappointing. Domperidone, a drug that increases the emptying of the stomach, helps over a third of people a great deal but may be ineffective in another third.

Most people find dysmotility disturbing but not incapacitating. It does not lead to more serious problems and usually gets better with time.

CROHN'S DISEASE

Crohn's disease can easily be mistaken for IBS and vice versa. In Crohn's disease, there is lasting inflammation within the gastro-intestinal tract, causing pain, diarrhoea, weight loss and sometimes obstruction or perforation of the bowel, which needs surgery. It can be a very serious disease, but in its milder forms physical examination and blood tests are normal, and the symptoms can be identical to those of IBS.

Crohn's disease can affect any part of the gut from the mouth to the anus. However, it most commonly affects the terminal ileum. This is the last part of the small bowel where it joins the large bowel in the right lower corner of the abdomen – the right iliac fossa (see Figure 5.3 and also Figure 1.1). Pain at this site is therefore common in Crohn's disease, but it is also the most common site of IBS pain. Mild Crohn's disease of the terminal ileum may show up with

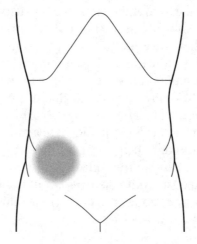

Figure 5.3 Pain in the right iliac fossa. This is the most frequent site of irritable bowel syndrome pain, but appendicitis, Crohn's disease and constipation all cause pain here too.

intermittent spasmodic pain in the right lower corner, sometimes with a disordered bowel habit. It can be indistinguishable from IBS.

Even with the usual tests such as a colonoscopy (putting a tube with a camera on up into the colon) to look at the large bowel, and a barium follow-through (swallowing a barium meal and taking X-rays while it is passing through the gut) to visualise the small bowel, Crohn's disease in just a small segment of bowel can be missed. In time, the Crohn's disease progresses and becomes more obvious. Weight loss, anaemia and a tender lump (your doctor may call it a 'mass') in the right lower area of the abdomen all suggest that something other than IBS is going on, and this should be investigated further. It can, however, take time – months or even years – before the true diagnosis becomes apparent.

Even once the Crohn's disease has been diagnosed and treated, the diagnostic problem recurs. IBS frequently occurs in bowel that has been inflamed. As a result, it can be unclear whether residual or recurrent symptoms are due to ongoing inflammation or to IBS that is also there. It is often a matter of judgement, and, as in many conditions, the doctor may need to try several treatments to see which works before being able to be more sure about the diagnosis.

APPENDICITIS

Acute appendicitis

Appendicitis is another cause of pain in the right lower corner of the abdomen (Figure 5.3), the most common site of IBS pain. The initial symptoms of appendicitis are vague and not specific to this condition. People report feeling unwell and being off their food. To start with, the pain is usually in the middle of the abdomen and may even occur in the upper abdomen. There is often nausea and vomiting, and people may suspect an upset stomach. The pain becomes worse when the infection spreads through the full thickness of the appendix wall. The pain then localises to where the appendix is, in the right lower corner. This process usually takes 24–48 hours.

Chronic or recurrent appendicitis

The concept of chronic appendicitis, sometimes called a 'grumbling appendix', as a cause of ongoing or intermittent right lower quadrant pain had been discredited because many people had had an appendicectomy (a removal of their appendix) without their symptoms improving. However, some people being admitted to hospital with acute appendicitis do describe previous episodes of pain that were the same as their current pain in all ways except its severity. In more recent surveys involving over 3600 appendicectomies, an average of 1.1% (range 0.01–3%) of people had had symptoms for at least 2 weeks before coming into hospital with more obvious appendicitis. When the removed appendix was examined, chronic appendicitis, as opposed to the usual acute appendicitis, was confirmed.

The concept of recurrent appendicitis is gradually being accepted, but many doctors still believe that similar prior episodes of abdominal pain make the diagnosis of appendicitis unlikely. So the very existence of recurrent and chronic appendicitis is still being debated.

ULCERATIVE COLITIS

In ulcerative colitis, the inflammation is confined to the large bowel and usually begins in the rectum and the lower bowel on the left side of the abdomen. It can cause diarrhoea and pain that comes in spasms in the left lower corner of the abdomen – the left iliac fossa (Figure 5.4). This is a common site for pain in IBS, so mild ulcerative colitis can initially be misdiagnosed as IBS.

However, there is usually, except in its mildest forms, some bleeding from the inflamed bowel with ulcerative colitis. Bleeding is not seen in IBS, except when there are piles (haemorrhoids) as well.

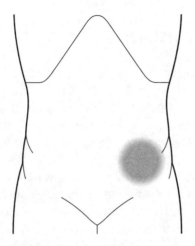

Figure 5.4 Pain in the left iliac fossa. Pain from irritable bowel syndrome and constipation frequently occurs here, but pain can also be caused by uncomplicated diverticular disease, diverticulitis and any infection or colitis affecting the lower part of the bowel.

Persistent bleeding, particularly if there are also loose stools and the person needs to get to the toilet quickly (urgency), suggests a problem in the rectum. The rectum is easily seen by sigmoidoscopy. As ulcerative colitis nearly always affects the rectum, the diagnosis is rarely missed.

The inflammation of ulcerative colitis can usually be successfully treated by medication, but unfortunately even when this inflammation has been completely suppressed, people may continue to have IBS-type symptoms. It can be difficult to know whether the loose stools, bloating and pain mean that the inflammation has come back or that the inflammation has caused an irritable bowel as well. In ulcerative colitis, the inflammation begins at the rectum, so, from a medical point of view, it is fairly straightforward to perform a limited examination of the rectum to assess how bad the inflammation is.

DIVERTICULAR DISEASE

The name 'diverticular disease' comes from the Latin word *diverticulum*, which means a 'small diversion from the normal path'. Many people have small pouches in their colons that bulge outward through weak spots, like an inner tube that pokes through weak places in a tyre. These weak spots occur between muscle bands where the blood vessels go into wall of the bowel. Each pouch is called a diverticulum. Several pouches are called diverticula. The condition of having these diverticula is called diverticulosis or diverticular disease. When the pouches become infected or inflamed, the condition is called diverticulitis.

Diverticular disease is so common as to be virtually a normal part of ageing. At least half of all 60-year-olds and most people over the age of 80 will have diverticular disease, predominantly affecting the left side of the bowel. Most will have minimal if any symptoms. About 10–25% of people with diverticulosis will get diverticulitis (infection involving a diverticulum), and about 5% will get bleeding from a diverticulum.

Uncomplicated diverticular disease

We do not know how many people have symptoms caused by uncomplicated diverticular disease (meaning that there is no infection or bleeding). Many people are entirely free of symptoms, whereas others will get symptoms that are indistinguishable from those of IBS. The most common symptoms are left-sided abdominal pain that comes in spasms, with a change in bowel habit, sometimes constipation and often pellet-like stools. Right-sided abdominal pain is unusual as 95% of diverticular disease is on the left. Eating extra fibre in the diet may help with symptoms more than it would in IBS.

Diverticulitis

Infection in a diverticulum has been described as a 'left-sided appendicitis'. Pain starts in the lower abdomen and tends to localise in the left lower corner (see Figure 5.4). There may be a lot of tenderness at the site of the pain, and movement may make the pain worse. Nausea, fever and a change in bowel habit are common. If the inflamed piece of colon is next to the bladder, there are also urinary symptoms. The symptoms tend to be continuous. If the diverticulitis is mild, it will settle over a week or two with or without antibiotics. More severe cases require admission to hospital and occasionally an operation.

ADHESIONS

Adhesions are abnormal bands of fibrous tissue inside the abdominal cavity. They can occur after abdominal surgery, or after any inflammation within the abdomen such as Crohn's disease or endometriosis (deposits of tissue similar to the tissue that lines the inside of the uterus, but occurring in the abdomen outside the uterus; see later in the chapter). Adhesions are responsible for the majority of bowel obstructions in the Western world. They also show up as chronic abdominal pain and infertility. Up to one third of people who have undergone open surgery on their abdomen are readmitted to hospital to deal with problems related to abdominal adhesions.

Small bowel obstruction from adhesions

The muscles of the small bowel continually contract and relax to propel digesting food onwards, so the small bowel is in a continual state of activity and motion (termed peristalsis). In doing this, it may become wrapped around or kinked across an adhesion. This causes the flow to become blocked at that point. The muscles react with

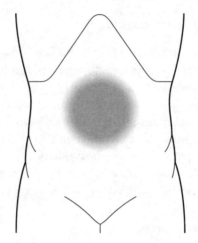

Figure 5.5 Central abdominal pain. Obstruction to the small or large bowel can produce severe, colicky pain at this site. Pain here can also be caused by disorders of the stomach, duodenum or aorta.

stronger and stronger contractions to try and force the food on. These contractions are felt as waves of severe pain that come and go in the middle of the abdomen (Figure 5.5). The accompanying nausea and vomiting are due to back-pressure.

It is usually necessary to go into hospital for pain relief and rehydration. The obstruction mostly resolves over 24–48 hours, but surgery is occasionally needed to cut the adhesions. This is only done if absolutely necessary as it can cause even more adhesions.

Occasionally, the obstruction to the small bowel is incomplete, and the pain and vomiting less severe. People with this problem learn that if they avoid food, and just drink for 24 hours, the problem will settle without having to go into hospital. Such episodes generally occur very intermittently every few weeks, months or years. Between them, bowel function is normal, unlike IBS, which tends to have some symptoms on most days.

Chronic pain from adhesions

Ongoing pain can also be caused by adhesions if they exert an abnormal pull on organs in the abdomen, or if nerves become trapped within them. This problem is difficult to diagnose as there are no abnormal physical signs, blood tests or scans. It can be distinguished from IBS because there are usually no other signs of abnormal bowel function. There is pain but no bloating, diarrhoea, constipation or abnormal stools.

RENAL COLIC

This is a pain caused by a sudden obstruction to the flow of urine from one kidney as a result of a stone getting stuck in the tube leading from the kidney to the bladder (the ureter) or just inside the kidney. The pain occurs only on the side with the obstruction (Figure 5.6). The usual course is for the pain to begin in the loin, in the side

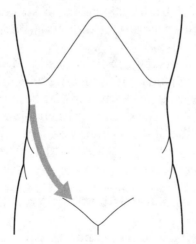

Figure 5.6 Renal colic on the right side. The arrow shows the direction the pain spreads in.

or in the upper abdomen, and travel down to the lower abdomen. It may spread into the pubic region, or into the penis or testicles in men. It occurs in waves and can be very severe. There is often also nausea and vomiting. Once the stone has passed, the pain goes away, and it only returns if the ureter is obstructed again by another stone. Between episodes, there are no symptoms. Bowel habit is not usually disturbed, except possibly by constipation from analgesics the person has taken to help the pain.

SLIPPING RIB SYNDROME

The slipping rib syndrome, sometimes also called costochondritis, may be caused by excessive movement of the front end of the costal cartilage. This is the cartilage that attaches the rib to the breastbone (sternum). It is usually the tenth rib that causes pain because, unlike ribs one to seven, which attach to the sternum, the eighth, ninth and tenth ribs are attached at the back to each other by loose, fibrous tissue. This means that there is more movement, but there is also a greater likelihood of trauma. Slipping rib syndrome is also more likely to occur in the lower ribs because the blood supply to the cartilage and ligaments is poor.

Costochondritis is usually easily recognised because people can point to localised pain and tenderness in the lower chest. Occasionally, however, they feel their pain to be more in the abdomen and just under the ribs. The doctor will then initially look for a problem in the abdomen, but the diagnosis is helped by the fact that the pain is not related to eating but is worse with breathing or movement.

FUNCTIONAL ABDOMINAL PAIN SYNDROME

Functional abdominal pain syndrome (also called chronic idiopathic abdominal pain or chronic functional abdominal pain) is fortunately uncommon. It is a severe pain that occurs daily and disturbs normal daily activities. Unlike IBS, the pain is not related to bowel function. Moreover, it can last into the night and disturb sleep, which is unusual with IBS. There are often underlying psychological problems, which the doctor can see but the person may not be aware of so keeps trying to discover a physical cause for the pain. The cause of this syndrome is unknown.

WHAT SHOULD MAKE ME WORRY ABOUT CANCER?

Cancer of the stomach

Doctors recognise what are called 'alarm symptoms', which suggest a serious condition. These include anaemia caused by iron deficiency, weight loss, difficulty swallowing, persistent vomiting or bleeding. Bleeding from the stomach appears as blood in the vomit, or as a melaena stool (a shiny black, loose stool, like tar, composed of partly digested blood). But even in patients with these symptoms, cancer is found in fewer than 10% of cases. Stomach cancer is rare under the age of 50.

Cancer of the bowel

A change in the bowel habit to looser, more frequent stools that lasts for more than a few weeks may be the first sign of bowel cancer. People with this symptom, especially if they are over the age of 50 (as bowel cancer is rare under the age of 50) will usually need an investigation of their bowel; this will usually involve a colonoscopy (examination using a tube with a miniature camera) or a barium enema (which shows up the bowel on an X-ray). Anaemia due to iron deficiency, weight loss and bleeding from the back passage are also worrying symptoms that need looking into. Again, most people with such symptoms do not turn out to have cancer. Pain without any of the other above symptoms is unusual in early cancer.

Cancer of the pancreas

The symptoms of cancer of the pancreas are very similar to those of chronic pancreatitis. Pain in the upper abdomen that spreads to the back, weight loss and diarrhoea are typical symptoms. Sometimes none of these symptoms occurs and the first sign of the disease is jaundice.

ENDOMETRIOSIS

Endometriosis is a puzzling disease affecting women in their reproductive years. The name comes from the word 'endometrium', which is the tissue that lines the inside of the womb (uterus) and builds up and sheds each month in the menstrual cycle. In endometriosis, tissue like the endometrium is found outside the uterus, in other areas of the body. In these places, it also builds up each month and then bleeds at menstruation. The bleeding irritates and inflames adjoining tissues. It can cause pain and other symptoms associated with menstruation.

Endometriosis is a common finding during operations for other problems, so most of the time it probably causes no symptoms at all. It is, however, also known as a 'great mimicker', and if your symptoms are very closely associated with your periods, endometriosis should be considered. It is usually diagnosed by a laparoscopy, a small operation in which a telescope is placed into the abdominal cavity.

MEDICALLY UNEXPLAINED ABDOMINAL PAIN

What do you mean by 'medically unexplained'?

This means that the symptom or symptoms do not fit any of the recognised medical conditions.

Does that mean that it's all in the mind?

That is not a phrase we currently use. People readily accept that physical illness can cause psychological symptoms such as anxiety, depression and fatigue, and there is no stigma attached to this. It is also common for psychological distress to manifest as physical symptoms, for example a tension headache. Today, we recognise a psychological and a physical component to all illnesses.

But you're saying that there's no physical explanation for my pain! Therefore you must be implying a mental explanation! Do you mean I'm mad?

In a few people, there may be a psychological problem underlying their pain, but that is *not* what is being implied when doctors cannot find a physical explanation for a pain.

There may not be a physical explanation for a headache. No brain tumour, no hangover, nothing wrong with the eyes. It may or may not be associated with stress, and it may or may not be a tension headache. Calling it such doesn't imply that the pain isn't real, nor does it suggest any form of 'madness'.

You could think of your pain as the equivalent of a tension headache in your abdomen.

I am not stressed or depressed. I sometimes get upset, angry and frustrated by this pain that nobody will do anything about. I'm fed up with being fobbed off with another scan, a different painkiller or another suggestion that I see a shrink. Why can't you find out what's causing it and give me the right treatment?

Unfortunately, modern medicine has its limitations. If you have seen a number of doctors and had the relevant tests, and your symptoms have not changed significantly over a long time, it is unlikely that any doctor will discover a precise diagnosis or a simple cure for you.

We all want a 'magic bullet' to sort out the cause of any illness, once and for all. Sadly, that is not always or even usually possible. If tests and treatments aren't being any help, you may gain more by approaching things from a different direction, for example working on coping strategies or relaxation therapies (see Chapter 11).

But I am in pain. The pain is real. Something physical must be wrong.

Unfortunately, this isn't necessarily the case. Most people's concept of pain comes from the experience of minor injury, which we encounter all the time. A twisted ankle hurts. A cut on the finger hurts – and the bigger the cut, the more it hurts. We see the pain as representing physical damage. The worse the pain, the worse the damage.

But this concept is misleading. For starters, it isn't even true of minor physical injuries. How much something hurts often depends on how much attention we pay to it. If we are distracted by other activities, we can ignore an injury. For example, footballers play on after a little dab from the physiotherapist's sponge. Wouldn't it be great if that sponge were available on the NHS? And what about badly wounded soldiers carrying on with apparently no pain? Yet at other times we can be disabled by headaches, or tummy aches, or back pain, when there is no discernable physical damage for anyone to see. The severity of pain is not proportional to physical damage.

I feel embarrassed that, after stridently complaining about my pain, nothing abnormal was found in any of the tests.

This is actually quite common, so don't feel embarrassed. There is no stigma attached to having symptoms without physical signs, or test results that don't show anything. Contrary to popular perception, there is often no relationship between the severity of the symptoms and the seriousness of the underlying disease.

If my tests are normal, will my doctor think that I have wasted his time?

Not at all. Most of the tests we perform today give normal results. This reflects the increasing availability of tests and our increasing inability to tolerate uncertainty.

On the one hand, it can be argued that when symptoms have occurred for a long time they are unlikely to represent serious disease, and that tests to confirm that there is nothing amiss are unnecessary. On the other hand, if symptoms have persisted for a long time, they may well persist for a still longer time, and the sooner you know that there is nothing there, the easier the symptoms will be to deal with.

How is it that our perception of pain can so inaccurately represent what's actually happening?

Our body is full of sensors that continually feed information to our central nervous system. These signals are processed and modified in the spinal cord and brain. Only a small proportion of the sensory signals generated actually reach our consciousness: most of the information received is processed subconsciously. When signals denoting pain reach the spinal cord, they compete with signals relaying sensation. So, if you cut your finger, it hurts less if you shake your hand or place it under a cold tap. This is also the principle behind TENS (transcutaneous electrical nerve stimulation), in which sensations produced by electrical stimulation reduce pain by competing with the pain signal at the spinal cord.

The signal can also be amplified or dampened down by nerve pathways coming down from the brain through the spinal cord. It is thought, for example, that stress or psychological distress can cause signals from the brain to amplify the pain signals coming into the spinal cord. So a signal that would previously have denoted a minor disturbance, or even normal function, and might not even have been registered consciously, now enters consciousness as pain.

I didn't understand that. Can you give me an analogy?

Imagine playing your favourite music CD in your state-of-the-art hi-fi. The music is beautiful. You go to the kitchen for a cup of tea, and your young child plays with the controls on the hi-fi. When you come back, the music is awful! Is there something wrong with the hi-fi, or is it the CD? No, it's to do with the way the knobs on the hi-fi are set – a signalling problem, if you like, between the CD and the speakers. How this happens in the human body is gradually being worked out. With IBS, you can read bowel for hi-fi, food for CD, and spinal cord plus lower brain for hi-fi controls.

I still don't want to see a shrink.

There are some people who would jump at the chance to have an intelligent and knowledgeable person help them to understand themselves and their reactions to the world around them. In some cultures, in fact, seeing a psychologist or psychiatrist is normal behaviour for normal people – the intellectual's equivalent of a 'lifestyle guru'. But it is expensive and time-consuming too. There are simpler alternatives you can try if you prefer, including hypnosis, meditation and other relaxation therapies (see Chapter 11).

I don't want to take antidepressants. I'm not depressed.

I can understand how you feel. Some people feel embarrassed even by the suggestion of antidepressants. In the past, when antidepressants were relatively ineffective and full of side effects, they were reserved for really desperate cases. Taking an antidepressant labelled people as severely, even hopelessly, depressed. With the introduction of the tricyclic antidepressants, and more recently the SSRIs (see Chapter 4), this perception has changed. Antidepressants are necessary for some people in the way in which medication for blood pressure is necessary for others. Certain antidepressants are frequently used for ongoing pain, whatever its cause. They are used for back pain, cancer pain, IBS and unexplained pain.

These medicines are often effective at very low doses. For example, the antidepressant amitriptyline is commonly used for pain at a dose of 10–40 mg a day, whereas the dose for depression is higher, at 75–150 mg per day. In the context of pain, antidepressants are not used to cheer people up and will work equally well whether or not the person is depressed. Moreover, the smaller dose means minimal if any side effects. Antidepressants are thought to work by altering processing of the pain signals in the spinal cord, but no one knows exactly how. Antidepressants take about 4 weeks to help depressed patients but can help immediately in pain syndromes. Some people take low-dose amitriptyline on and off depending on the severity of their pain.

It's also worth considering that you might just be depressed. Depression is an illness, not a stigma, and like all illnesses, it can present in atypical ways. It is possible for the physical symptoms of depression to outweigh the psychological symptoms. You may benefit from taking the full dose of a modern antidepressant; these are now effective, with minimal if any side effects. It could take about 1 month of treatment before you see any benefits, but years of suffering might be relieved.

If I am depressed, it's because of my illness. Depression is not the cause of my pain. Is there really any point in taking antidepressants?

You may have what is called a 'reactive depression'. This is when the depression follows a life event or events, and would not have occurred without that event. With support, most people can face life's crises, adjusting to their new circumstances. Hence, in most people, reactive depression tends to stop of its own accord.

But if you have ongoing ill health, especially when there has been no clear diagnosis or treatment, adjusting can be very difficult. Failing to adjust leads to a prolonged depression, and this depression itself makes adjustment more difficult. It is easy then to feel that any solution or help that's offered won't help. You can become trapped in a vicious circle. By lifting the depression, antidepressants can break this. You may still not have an explanation or a treatment for your original illness, and the uncertainty will still be there, but the symptoms will have less of an effect on your life.

> *I still don't want to take antidepressants. Is there anything else to try?*

Cognitive behavioural therapy is a short-term psychological treatment that is particularly suitable for specific, focused problems (see Chapter 11).

It is based on the assumption that 'thought intercedes between stimulus and emotion'. In other words, whatever is causing the initial pain provokes thoughts, assumptions or interpretations, which then lead to emotions. The emotions will interact with whatever has caused the reaction in the first place, amplifying it, making it worse, and so on into a vicious circle. For example, the pain may generate thoughts such as 'I've got cancer!', or 'I can't cope today', or 'Those doctors are bloody useless.' These thoughts generate negative emotions such as fear, hopelessness and anger, which in turn make the pain worse.

Cognitive behavioural therapy aims to understand the thought processes that the symptoms produce and how they can make things worse. It then aims to teach you to substitute more positive thoughts to break the circle of negative thoughts leading to negative emotions, leading to more symptoms.

> *Is this another way in which doctors try to blame what they don't understand on their patients? You don't understand my illness, you can't do anything about it, and that must be my fault! Isn't that what generations of doctors have done?*

I have some sympathy with this viewpoint. Since the dawn of history, people have reported symptoms that their doctors could not explain in terms of actual physical findings. The theories dreamed up to explain such symptoms in the past appear ludicrous today, and no doubt today's offerings will amuse future generations.

In the Middle Ages, for example, much was blamed on the uterus. In fact, the word 'hysteria' comes from the Latin *hystera*, meaning womb. The treatment of 'hysteria' centred on 'physical' treatments for the uterus, such as massaging the pelvic area, applying various creams and ointments to the female genitals, and even manual stimulation of the woman's genitals by the doctor to 'hysterical paroxysm', presumably orgasm! Indeed, the vibrator was originally developed as a medical treatment for hysteria. As these treatments didn't work, the word 'hysteria' came to mean symptoms caused by wild and uncontrollable emotion. The same thought process sometimes happens today too, but I think our explanations and treatments are more scientifically based and objectively tested than ever before.

More of a problem is some people's great focus on the mind–body problem. They are unable to perceive how the two interact. Any suggestion of a psychological component for their symptoms is utterly rejected and seen as an insult, when nothing could be further from the truth. This approach unfortunately means that they deny themselves a huge avenue of help and self-understanding.

I'm still worrying that my pain represents a cancer. Could the doctors have got it wrong?

No doctor or medical test is perfect. But for cancers to cause pain, they usually have to be large enough to obstruct the bowel or seriously disrupt an adjacent organ. And such large tumours are unlikely to be missed. In my experience, when people have pain, either the cancer is obvious or there is no cancer.

SUMMARY

■ Most abdominal conditions are recognised by the way in which people describe their symptoms. Doctors listen out for patterns of symptoms that suggest certain conditions and perform tests to confirm or deny their suspicions.

■ To make use of your doctor – and this book – it is vital to give a clear description of your pain especially in terms of:

◆ the site of the pain;

◆ its timing, how often it occurs and for how long;

◆ what makes it better or worse;

◆ associated symptoms such as nausea, vomiting, diarrhoea, constipation, weight loss or bleeding.

■ Pain does not necessarily mean physical damage or disease.

■ Pain caused by cancer is usually associated with other symptoms, especially weight loss.

6 | Bloating and wind

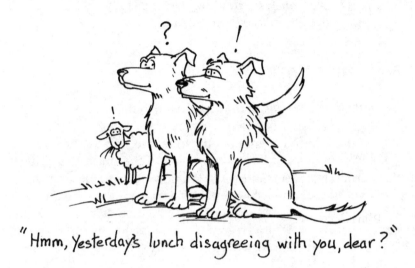

"Hmm, Yesterday's lunch disagreeing with you, dear?"

Bloating is one of the most common symptoms of irritable bowel syndrome (IBS), affecting more than 90% of people with IBS. For some individuals, the bloating is more disturbing than the disordered bowel habit, and more difficult to live with than the pain. In one survey, 60% of those with IBS reported bloating as their most bothersome symptom. It is more commonly associated with the constipation-predominant type of IBS, but relieving the constipation does not always relieve the bloating. Bloating and abdominal distension typically occur after meals, become progressively worse during the day and settle after a night's sleep.

It's worth remembering that about 30% of people without IBS will also experience bloating from time to time. It is more common in women and may be worse during their periods.

Most treatments for IBS are aimed at normalising the bowel habit and reducing the pain, but little is known about their effects on bloating. There are no specific treatments for bloating, and some doctors are not even sure that the abdominal distension really exists. In recent years, though, we have learned a lot more about gas production and transport in the intestine, and hopefully this distressing symptom will not be ignored in the future.

GAS IN THE BOWEL

Where does all the gas in the bowel come from?

Gas in the intestine comes mainly from two sources. First, we all inadvertently swallow air, even when we're not eating. This is called aerophagia. We can't avoid swallowing some air, but this is usually harmless. Eating slowly and swallowing only small amounts at a time during meals, not sucking hard sweets or chewing gum, and avoiding fizzy drinks is often recommended to reduce aerophagia, but this has not been rigorously tested and is usually disappointing in practice.

The other source of gas is the fermentation of food, especially undigested plant material in the large bowel, by bacteria in the gut. So the volume and constituents of the gas depend partly on the diet and partly on the number and type of bacteria in the bowel – what is called the 'bacterial flora'. Some carbon dioxide gas is also produced when acid from the stomach is neutralised by the alkali in the duodenum. But carbon dioxide is rapidly absorbed into the bloodstream and removed through the lungs, so this is not a major factor.

What is flatus made up of?

Much of the flatus is air that has been swallowed with the food and passed down the intestine. The carbon dioxide and oxygen in this air are mostly absorbed into the body, leaving the nitrogen behind. Some gas is also produced in the large bowel; this is mainly hydrogen and products of hydrogen such as hydrogen sulphide and methane.

Why does flatulence smell so bad?

The gases that make up flatus are mostly hydrogen, carbon dioxide and methane. Flatus smells obnoxious because of the breakdown of compounds containing sulphur. The main smelly gas in flatus is hydrogen sulphide (as in rotten eggs). Other malodorous gases include methanethiol and dimethyl sulphide.

It is likely that differences in the concentration of these gases are determined partly by the diet and partly by the bacterial flora (the bacteria that live in the gut). This is why the odour varies between individuals and why individuals can recognise the smell of their own flatus. Some foods, such as cabbage, eggs, onions and meat, contain more sulphur than others.

How much gas does the average person have in their intestine?

Not a lot – only about 200–400 ml, which is about 1–2 glassfuls.

And how much gas does an average person pass in a day?

There's a lot of variation between people, and even in the same person at different times, but about 200–2500 ml (between one-half and 5 pints) a day is normally produced.

I'm sure men seem to pass more flatus than women, and that it smells worse. Is this true?

This common belief has actually been studied in a small experiment. The flatus from women was found to have a greater concentration of hydrogen sulphide and was judged to have a worse odour. But men tended to pass greater volumes of flatus at a time, so overall there was no significant difference!

WHAT CAUSES BLOATING IN IBS?

Is bloating real? Does my tummy really distend through the day?

Some doctors believe that the bloating and distension of IBS are perceived rather than real. In other words, individuals feel discomfort in their abdomen, or are unhappy with what feels like a bloated abdomen, and misinterpret these feelings, believing their abdomen to be distended.

Many studies have looked at this question. The girth of the abdomen (the measurement all the way round) has been examined by simple measurement, by X-rays and by CT (computed tomography) scanning. All these studies confirmed a real increase in the abdominal circumference in people with IBS. Although there were considerable changes in these measurements over a 24-hour period, they usually increased after meals, were lowest during sleep and increased progressively during the day. Interestingly, the measured increase in girth was only poorly related to the severity of the symptoms that the person reported.

Is this bloating caused by gas?

Excess gas in the intestine is probably the main cause of bloating. It was previously thought that most of this gas was produced by the bacterial fermentation of plant material in the large bowel. However, recent studies suggest that it is gas in the small bowel that causes the problem (a question later in this chapter describes the experiment that was performed).

How does this gas get into the small bowel?

The small bowel is normally sterile, meaning that there are no bacteria, and the gas in it comes from swallowed air.

What happens if bacteria do get into the small bowel?

The small bowel leads into the large bowel (see Figure 1.1 in Chapter 1), but the two are separated by a valve called the ileo-caecal valve. This valve acts to stop the contents of the large bowel passing back into the small bowel. This is important because the large bowel is full of bacteria, whereas the small bowel is normally sterile. The valve is not fully effective, but bacteria entering the small bowel are normally rapidly flushed back into the large bowel.

However, bacteria from the large bowel sometimes manage to stay in the small bowel. This is called small bowel bacterial overgrowth. The infection does not usually cause fever or pain as the bacteria do not actually invade the wall of the bowel. They do, however, interfere with digestion. In severe cases, this results in diarrhoea and weight loss. It has been suggested that, in milder cases, the main symptom might be bloating due to the gas produced by these bacteria. So it is possible that small bowel bacterial overgrowth may be an important part of what causes IBS.

What happens to air in the small bowel?

This air is normally rapidly propelled down the small bowel. Gas is propelled much more rapidly than food and can pass through the entire length of the intestine in less than half an hour. But not all the air we swallow is passed out. The carbon dioxide is absorbed into the bloodstream and removed from the body via the lungs. Most of the oxygen is also absorbed, but some of it is used by the bacteria in the large bowel. The nitrogen, which forms 78% of the air, passes into the large bowel and then out of the body as flatus.

I've got IBS. Does this mean that I'm producing more gas?

Probably not, but no one really knows yet. Some studies show no increase in gas production, whereas others show a small increase. One study published in the medical journal *The Lancet* in

1998 showed that more hydrogen was produced in people with IBS compared with people without IBS eating the same diet. But the difference was small – 332 ml compared with 162 ml over 24 hours for the two groups. In terms of volume, this is just a glass of water and cannot account for any bloating. Moreover, when total gas production, including methane, was measured, there was no significant difference between those with and those without IBS.

But if people with IBS don't produce a lot more gas, why do they bloat?

The problem here is impaired transport of gas down the small intestine rather than too much gas being produced. Until recently, bloating and excess wind were thought to be a large bowel problem. But an elegant series of experiments on people with and without IBS by a group of doctors in Barcelona changed our understanding of how gas is handled in the intestine, and the causes of bloating.

These experiments involved gas (a mixture of oxygen, nitrogen and carbon dioxide) being continuously blown into the small intestine through a small tube passed down through the mouth. Within half an hour, the gas started to come out through the anus, and it was then collected and measured. The amount of gas retained ('trapped') in the intestine was then calculated as the difference between the volume of gas going into the tube in the mouth and the volume of gas collected from the anus. The people with IBS retained significantly more gas – over 400 ml after 2 hours. As a result, their abdominal girth increased by 7 mm, compared with just 1 mm in those without IBS. Moreover, over half of those with IBS experienced significant discomfort, whereas none of the other group did.

Further studies have shown that gas infused into the small bowel causes significantly more symptoms than a similar volume infused into the large bowel. Interestingly, there was the same degree of abdominal distension each time, but it was gas in the small bowel that proved uncomfortable.

It now seems clear that the uncomfortable bloating of IBS results from problems in the movement of gas down the small intestine, causing gas to be retained in the small intestine. This is in contrast to the previous, and still widely held, belief that bloating is caused by too much gas in the large bowel. The small intestine is only 2–3 centimetres wide, compared with 5 centimetres for the large intestine, so relatively smaller volumes of gas held in localised parts of the small intestine may be responsible for the uncomfortable feeling of 'trapped gas' that is so common in IBS.

Do we know why people with abdominal bloating have this problem with transport of intestinal gas?

There are a number of reflexes that help to control the intestine. Glucose (a type of sugar) entering the small bowel tends to speed up transport along the small intestine, whereas fat in the small intestine slows it down. This makes sense as fat is more difficult to digest than sugar so needs to stay in the intestine for longer. In one experiment, the researchers put gas along with fat into the small intestine. In all the subjects, some of the gas was retained because propulsion down the small intestine was slower. But significantly more gas was retained in individuals with IBS, suggesting that they had a stronger response to fat.

Another reflex that normally helps to keep things moving is triggered from the rectum: if the rectum is distended, gas moves more quickly down the small intestine. This reflex can be strong enough to counteract the slowing effect of fat. In one study, researchers put air bags into the rectums of people with and without IBS and inflated these so that they could just be felt. In people without IBS, inflating the air bag caused the gas to move more quickly down the small intestine. It also prevented a fat infusion delaying gas transport. But in people with IBS, rectal distension did not stop gas being retained. Unfortunately, we don't yet know why IBS impairs the reflex control of the intestine in this way.

FOOD AND BLOATING

Why do I feel bloated when I eat rich or fatty foods?

Fat is more difficult to digest than other foods. This may explain why there are normal reflexes that aim to slow the emptying of the stomach after a fatty meal, and to slow movement through the small intestine (see the previous question) – this allows more time for digestion. It is possible that these reflexes are exaggerated in people with IBS.

Which foods are most likely to make gas problems and bloating worse?

In a survey of 330 people with IBS, the foods most commonly reported to produce abdominal distension or gas problems were pizza, cabbage, onion, peas/beans, raw vegetables and deep-fried food.

When we look at the previous questions, we can see why fatty foods such pizza and fried foods might produce bloating. The common experience that high-fibre foods also cause bloating suggests that fermentation of fibre in the large bowel does indeed have a role.

Why could fibre in the diet make bloating worse?

The traditional view is that fibre passes largely undigested from the small intestine into the large intestine. There it is fermented by bacteria to produce gases such as hydrogen, hydrogen sulphide and methane. So the more fibre ingested, the more gas will be produced. But recent research strongly suggests that uncomfortable bloating is a consequence of gas retention in the small intestine (see earlier in the chapter), implying that fermentation of fibre can't fully explain the problem although it probably contributes.

Does eating fibre affect how quickly gas goes through the small intestine?

A high-fibre diet may slow the movement of gas, leading to gas retention and bloating.

The effect of a high-fibre diet on gas transit has only recently been examined. In a study from the USA involving ten people without IBS, gas was infused into the small intestine via a tube passed through the mouth. The gas was collected by another tube placed in the rectum. Each person was studied twice: once after a standard diet for 7 days, and once after the same diet had been supplemented by 30 g of a substance called psyllium each day. Psyllium (*Ispaghula* husk) is a form of fibre frequently recommended for IBS, usually in sachets containing 3.5 g, and the dose prescribed in the study was larger than the 10 g or so a day usually recommended for IBS.

Once the gas had begun to be infused in the experiment, there was a delay before gas appeared at the rectum. This delay showed the time taken for the gas to pass all the way down the intestine. After a normal diet, gas reached the rectum in an average of 19 minutes, but after the high-fibre diet it took 38 minutes. Moreover, after the high-fibre diet, almost 400 ml of the gas was trapped in the intestine, whereas after the standard diet there was no gas retention.

It is not clear why fibre in the form of psyllium slows gas transit through the intestine. It is possible that the increased bulk of the fibre forms a mechanical obstruction to the flow of gas. Or the fibre may hold onto the gas in the same way in which it retains water in the stool.

Another intriguing possibility involves the gas methane. About 70% of us have bacteria in our bowel that can ferment fibre to methane. Some of this methane is absorbed into the bloodstream and widely distributed throughout the body, finally being excreted by the lungs. A surprising finding is that methane seems to slow the intestine down, an effect studied so far only in dogs. Intriguingly, in humans, excess methane measured in the breath has been associated with constipation.

If I eat more fibre, will it make my bloating better?

Bloating is most frequently associated with the constipation-predominant form of IBS. Some people find taking extra fibre a great help in regulating their bowel and relieving their constipation. And often, but not always, relief of the constipation helps with the bloating. It may be worth trying to increase the fibre content of your diet for a few weeks. Bear in mind that extra fibre may initially make the bloating worse, before relief of the constipation improves it. (Chapter 7 provides some more information on constipation.)

Could anything else cause the bloating?

Another explanation for bloating has been termed 'abdominal proptosis'. In this, the abdominal muscles fail to tighten up in response to a full intestine after a meal. This can combine with an excess curvature of the lumbar spine (the lower back). The abdomen therefore gets pushed out, making it look distended. Little evidence has been published to support this explanation, but there is no reason why it should not to be a contributory cause for bloating in some people. It's possible that strengthening your abdominal muscles with exercise such as sit-ups may help.

PROBLEMS AND SOLUTIONS

I know that some people with cancer or cirrhosis of the liver can get very bloated because their abdomen fills with fluid. How can I know if my bloating is caused by fluid?

There is normally very little if any fluid between the internal organs and the abdominal wall. When fluid does accumulate here, it is called free fluid or ascites. This fluid is shifted by gravity, and the distension caused by ascites can be seen to affect the lower part of the abdomen when the individual is standing, and the sides when he or she is lying down. Ascites comes and goes very slowly over days and weeks. By contrast, the bloating of IBS comes on rapidly after meals or develops through the day. It also resolves after a night's sleep. So if you are not bloated when you wake up, you can be sure that fluid is not accumulating in your abdomen.

Can constipation make me bloated?

A large bowel heavily loaded with stool can certainly cause abdominal distension. Such distension will not resolve with a night's sleep. The diagnosis of constipation is usually obvious to everyone, but occasionally an abdominal X-ray is necessary to assess it. (For more information on constipation, see Chapter 7.)

What can I do to stop passing all this wind?

Passing wind is normal and unavoidable! Healthy people pass flatus an average of 14 times a day, with a volume of 25–100 ml (up to half a glassful) each time. You should not, in fact, try to hold it in as there is some evidence that voluntarily holding onto the wind slows down gas transit in the intestine. And this may increase bloating. It's healthy just to let the wind pass.

In that case, can I do anything to reduce the volume of wind that I pass?

Eat slowly and chew well so as to swallow less air. Eat less fibre, especially less of the highly fermentable foods such as beans, brussel sprouts, cabbage, onions, fruit juice in some people, and cereals. If you suspect that a particular food is causing your flatulence or bloating, you can test your suspicion by avoiding it for a few days to a week. If avoiding a food works, it's worth confirming the link by eating the food again. Many people make associations between certain foods and symptoms that are not borne out on retesting, and it would be a shame to limit your diet for nothing. (For more information on food intolerance, see Chapter 9.)

The popular laxative lactulose is also a common cause of wind.

Is there anything I can do about the smell I feel I'm making?

Medicinal ('activated') charcoal taken with meals will absorb aromatic gases such as hydrogen sulphide, causing the smell of the flatus to diminish or even go away all together. The charcoal does not work straight away, as it has to pass through the large bowel to have an effect. You will see it turn your stool dark. Some people take charcoal on a regular basis. Others take it for a few days before a social event or if they are about to have a meal they feel will cause them trouble. Charcoal is available without prescription from chemists and health food shops as tablets or capsules.

The indigestion remedy bismuth subsalicylate (Pepto-Bismol) can also reduce the smell by absorbing any hydrogen sulphide. It's available from the chemist without prescription.

Some people find that taking peppermint oil capsules helps to make the smell of their flatulence less unpleasant.

Charcoal-lined cushions, underwear made from carbon fibre, and charcoal panty liners to absorb the gases are available but are expensive.

What is the best way of masking the smell?

Striking a match is the simplest method. Some of the gas will burn (not visibly) and the whiff of smoke will effectively mask any remaining smell; it's easy to keep a small box of matches with you. Perfume or deodorant sprays are a more expensive alternative to mask the smell.

What is simethicone?

Simethicone is a non-prescription drug that acts on the surface of bubbles by reducing the surface tension, causing the bubbles to break up. It causes gas bubbles to break and join together, forming larger bubbles. Why this should improve symptoms is unclear, but it is widely promoted for 'gas' problems in IBS. It is available without prescription but tends to be more expensive than charcoal. In my experience, charcoal works better but simethicone is more palatable.

Is there any truth in the traditional advice that taking a walk after meals helps the food to digest?

Interestingly, there is evidence that gas moves more quickly down the small intestine if you are standing up rather than lying down. This comes from a small study on volunteers without IBS, but it does suggest that bloating may be diminished by keeping upright after meals. Whether walking itself has an effect is not known, but do try it as it might help you.

Are there any medicines that can help with bloating?

There are no medications specifically recommended for bloating. Many of the medicines that help with pain, constipation or diarrhoea do not help the bloating, but there are a few drugs you can try.

Domperidone (Motilium) is often tried to help bloating. It is actually marketed as an antiemetic (a medicine to stop you being sick) and is useful in nausea from any cause. It works by increasing peristalsis (the co-ordinated contractions of the gut that propel the contents forwards), mainly in the stomach and small intestine. Domperidone does not cross into the brain and is very safe. It therefore sounds ideal for disorders caused by slow movement through the stomach and small intestine. But studies of domperidone in IBS have produced disappointing results, with no great benefit compared with a placebo (dummy) treatment.

In practice, I feel that about a third of patients who use it get significant benefit. It is available without prescription in the UK as Motilium but is fairly expensive to buy over the counter. If fullness after meals is a problem for you, it may be worth asking your doctor for a prescription.

I sometimes feel like sticking a needle into my belly to let all the air out. I know that's silly, but what would actually happen?

It's certainly tempting to burst the balloon, but that's not what would happen! Even if the needle did penetrate a part of the bowel containing gas, it is not under such high pressure that it would vent to the outside. Moreover, the contraction of the gut muscles effectively separates the bowel into different compartments, so that even if you drained one part of gas, the rest would remain. Doctors often insert needles through the abdominal wall to drain fluid from within the abdominal cavity. Occasionally, we get it wrong and there is no fluid actually there. In such circumstances, the needle may penetrate the bowel wall – then we may be able to aspirate a little air, but otherwise nothing very much happens.

What can I do to prevent or reduce the bloating I feel?

Although our understanding of bloating has improved, our treatments still have a long way to go. All we can do is infer from our current knowledge that some changes in diet and lifestyle might help. I usually suggest the following:

1. Eat slowly and carefully, and chew well to avoid swallowing air.

2. Eat low-fat, high-carbohydrate foods. We saw in an earlier question that fat in the small bowel slows the transit of gas, whereas sugar speeds it up.

3. Eat less fibre. Fibre slows the movement of gas and is fermented to produce yet more gas.

④ If you become constipated, use 'stimulant' laxatives like senna rather than those called 'osmotic' laxatives, such as lactulose.

⑤ Exercise to tighten your abdominal muscles and lose weight.

⑥ Try medicinal ('activated') charcoal.

⑦ Try domperidone.

⑧ Buy loose-fitting clothes to make you feel more comfortable.

⑨ Try a combination of things as different things suit different people.

SUMMARY

■ IBS really does cause bloating.

■ The bloating gets worse during the day and settles at night.

■ It is mostly due to air retained in the small bowel.

■ Air in the small bowel comes mostly from air swallowed with food.

■ Fibre in the diet usually makes bloating worse.

■ The bloating is occasionally due to constipation.

■ A fatty meal may make the bloating worse.

■ Foods reported to produce most gas problems include pizza, cabbage, onion, peas/beans, raw vegetables and deep-fried food.

■ Medicinal (activated) charcoal is probably the best treatment to reduce the smell of flatulence. Peppermint oil can improve the aroma.

■ Bloating remains one of the most difficult symptoms to treat, but our increasing understanding of its underlying mechanisms will hopefully lead to better treatments in the future.

7 | CONSTIPATION

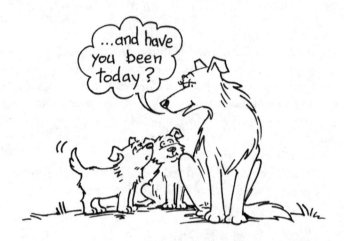

People say they have constipation if they think that they defecate too infrequently or with too much effort, if their stools are too hard or too small, if defecation is painful, or if they feel that they haven't emptied their rectum completely. This can also be confused by the fact that what is constipation to one person may be the usual situation for another.

Today, people and their doctors are more concerned with discomfort than with the number of stools passed or their size and shape, but a century ago constipation was big business. It was considered to be the scourge of civilisation, the source of many diseases and an explanation for all those symptoms that couldn't be explained by anything else. People became obsessed with keeping their bowels regularly cleared. Laxative sales took off, and high fibre-products were highly promoted. As a house officer in Plymouth when I qualified over 20 years ago, we would first do a ward round of the patients and then one of their stools – all carefully saved for our inspection by the nurses! Stools were serious stuff, and lectures on the evils of a low-fibre diet were commonplace.

But somehow constipation was already falling off its pedestal as the disease of civilisation. Perhaps it was the failure of laxatives to transform lives, the need for a more sophisticated diagnosis or indeed a greater understanding of the links between the mind and the gut. And so the concept of the irritable bowel syndrome (IBS) evolved and became popular. Today, people more readily admit to an irritable bowel and can accept it, probably correctly, as an explanation of many of their symptoms.

Constipation remains a common problem. Most of us will become constipated from time to time, often for no clearly definable reason. Some of us will have constipation as part of the constellation of symptoms that form IBS. About a third of people with IBS have constipation as one of their main problems (described as IBS-C).

IS MY BOWEL HABIT NORMAL?

Is there any right number of times to open my bowels each day?

About 50% of people open their bowel once a day, and most people open their bowel at least three times a week. But there is a wide variation among people such that it is perfectly normal for some people to open their bowels several times a day, whereas others are comfortable with just one bowel motion a week. There is no hard and fast rule. You should listen to the 'call to stool' from your bowel and go as often as you need to.

I have heard that it is abnormal to open the bowels more than three times per day, or less than three times per week. It this so?

These are definitions used in studies, surveys and clinical guidelines. They suggest that something may be wrong, such as IBS, or that the individual is at one or other extreme of the normal range.

Should I try and go regularly?

No, you don't need to do this. Most people have an irregular pattern and do not have bowel movements every day or even the same number of bowel movements each day.

What should my stool look like, and what consistency should it be?

The consistency and shape of your stool may be a better guide to how fast or slow your bowel is than the number of times that you go. Passing separate hard lumps, like nuts, or a lumpy sausage (Figure 7.1) suggests that your bowel may be slow or constipated. This is because the longer a stool remains in the bowel, the more water is absorbed from it and the harder it becomes. However, it

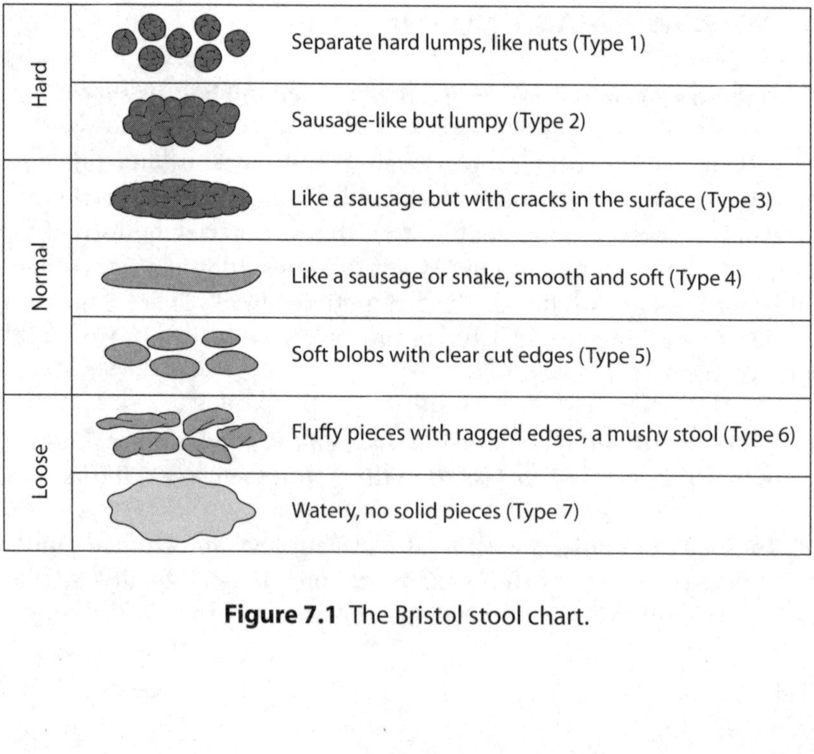

Hard		Separate hard lumps, like nuts (Type 1)
		Sausage-like but lumpy (Type 2)
Normal		Like a sausage but with cracks in the surface (Type 3)
		Like a sausage or snake, smooth and soft (Type 4)
		Soft blobs with clear cut edges (Type 5)
Loose		Fluffy pieces with ragged edges, a mushy stool (Type 6)
		Watery, no solid pieces (Type 7)

Figure 7.1 The Bristol stool chart.

doesn't matter what your stool looks like or what consistency it has as long as you are comfortable. If the stool is so hard that you frequently have to strain, you are constipated. Mucus (slime) passing along with the stool is normal in some people but is more common in people with an irritable bowel.

When should I worry about what my stool looks like?

A yellow, particularly foul-smelling stool that is loose, tends to float and is difficult to flush away is called steatorrhoea. It suggests that the digestion and absorption of food, especially fat, is impaired. You should consult your family doctor if you suspect that you are getting steatorrhoea.

A tarry black, loose and shiny stool with a different smell is called melaena. This indicates bleeding from high in the gastrointestinal tract, usually the stomach or duodenum (see Figure 1.1). Blood passing through the gut becomes partially digested, losing its red colour and turning a shiny black. Blood in the gut acts as a laxative so the stool is loose. When the bleeding is still going on, the stool is liquid and shiny black. When the bleeding has stopped and previously bled blood is coming out, the stool loses its shine but remains black. If you think that you have melaena, you should phone your family doctor as you may need admission to hospital.

Bright red blood, described by doctors as 'fresh' blood, usually comes from the lower parts of the gastrointestinal tract. It looks like blood because there has not been time for any digestion to take place. If there is blood just on the toilet paper, or on an otherwise usual-looking stool, the blood is likely to be coming from the anus or the rectum. Commonly, this is from haemorrhoids, which are large rectal veins, but it can be due to polyps (small mushroom-like growths, usually benign) or tumours (larger growths, sometimes malignant and sometimes benign) and should be taken seriously, especially in people over the age of 50. If there is fresh blood mixed in with the stool, the site of the bleeding is probably above the rectum but within about 40 centimetres (16 inches) of the anus. Common causes include inflammatory bowel disease, polyps, tumours and diverticular disease (see Chapter 5).

This symptom should be investigated at any age, usually with a flexible sigmoidoscopy (see Chapter 13 for more on this technique). If you are passing small amounts of blood (small specks to several teaspoons), make an appointment with your family doctor. If you are passing cupfuls of blood, phone your doctor as you may need admission to hospital.

Sometimes I get some slime coming out with my stool. Does that mean that I have IBS?

Mucus (slime) is common in IBS and in other conditions affecting the bowel. But it can also occur in those who do not have IBS. It suggests that the rectum is irritated, much as the nose can be irritated by a cold or an allergy. But just as you can get mucus from the nose without having anything wrong, mucus from the rectum can be normal in some people.

I only open my bowels once or twice a week. I'm perfectly happy with this, but am I doing myself any long-term harm by not going more regularly?

If you are comfortable, it does not matter how infrequently your bowels are open.

There was a theory, which some people still believe, that not clearing the bowel frequently would cause ill-health in both the short and the long term. This theory, called 'autointoxication', suggested that the rotting waste in the bowel produced toxins that could be absorbed to produce disease. This idea started in ancient Egyptian times and became the standard medical view in the 19th century. As a popular American health manual warned in the 1850s, 'daily evacuation of the bowels is of the utmost importance to the maintenance of health'. Without this daily movement, 'the entire system will become deranged and corrupted'! Many symptoms were blamed on constipation, including fatigue, poor sleep, headaches, poor memory, bad breath, a coated tongue, depression, aching muscles and joints, hair loss and impotence. It was felt to be the cause of colon cancer and even heart disease.

Processed foods were blamed then, as they are today. 'The whiter your bread, the sooner you're dead' is a saying attributed to the famous surgeon Sir William Arbuthnot Lane, who popularised a treatment for constipation that involved removing the large bowel. The cereal All-Bran was introduced in the early 1900s precisely to combat this autointoxication, as were any number of other bran cereals; stimulant laxatives were widely used, and colonic irrigation was born.

A number of experimental studies in the 1910s cast doubt on the idea of bowel toxins getting into the circulation, so autointoxication as a theory slowly faded away during the 1920s. But in the 1970s, the theory was revived by the English surgeon Dennis Burkitt. When he was in Uganda, he noticed that Africans produced several times more faeces than Westernised people did. In addition, their faeces were soft and produced with virtually no discomfort, again in contrast to Westernised people. Burkitt then suggested that one major cause of Western disease was eating large amounts of refined carbohydrates, which contain little dietary fibre. Burkitt's book *Don't Forget Fibre in your Diet*, published in 1979, spurred a popular revolution in diet.

Today, the causes of various diseases and how they may relate to our diet are closely studied in large studies over several countries. It seems that our longer-term health is improved by dietary fibre and that constipation may increase the risk of diverticular disease (see Chapter 5) and bowel cancer. But there is no evidence for 'autointoxication' as a cause of chronic fatigue, headaches, muscle pains or any of the other myriad symptoms we may develop. What is also clear is the wide variation in normal function between healthy people. So after all this information, the answer is quite short – if you are comfortable with your current bowel habit, you do not need to make any changes.

Should I set aside a specific time to open my bowels?

The bowel tends to be more active in the morning, and distension of the stomach following breakfast may also stimulate the bowel. If that describes you, you would be wise to allow enough time in the morning to attend to your bowel. If you keep suppressing the need to go to the toilet, the urge to defecate may get weaker, and this is one way in which people can become constipated.

Is there any best position to sit on the toilet?

When a person is standing up, there is an angle of about 90 degrees between the rectum and the anal canal. This is there to help with continence, that is, to help keep the faeces in during our normal activities. So, to defecate successfully, the anal canal and rec-

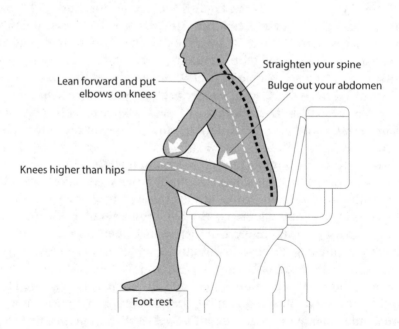

Lean forward and put elbows on knees

Straighten your spine

Bulge out your abdomen

Knees higher than hips

Foot rest

Figure 7.2 The best position to sit on the toilet.

tum must be in as straight a line as possible. This is achieved by bending at the hips. The ideal is a squatting position, but sitting down is more comfortable.

When you are sitting on the toilet, the best position is to place your elbows on your knees, keep your back straight, push your belly out, pretend to blow up a balloon so as to increase the pressure in your chest and abdomen and bear down (Figure 7.2). Lifting your feet off the ground will also help.

So are squatting toilets better?

Squatting does make defecation easier, so if you have problems passing stool a squatting toilet may be better. However, in cultures where this is the norm, haemorrhoids are more common.

WHY DO I GET CONSTIPATED?

What causes constipation?

When constipation is the main symptom, the underlying problem is usually IBS or what is called idiopathic constipation (which means constipation without an obvious cause).

There are many causes of constipation – the main ones are listed in Table 7.1. It is often impossible for any doctor to give a precise explanation of why a particular person has become constipated. There may be a multitude of possible factors, a combination of factors or even no explanation at all. The distinction between idiopathic (unknown aetiology) constipation and constipation-predominant IBS is also unclear. It's rare for cancer to show up with constipation as its main symptom.

It is a widely held belief that the main cause of constipation is insufficient dietary fibre, but this belief is not supported by research studies. Although more fibre in the diet will help constipation, people who are constipated do not actually eat less fibre than those who are not. Neither do they drink less fluid, and drinking more fluid doesn't usually help. The list in Table 7.1 is not complete as many conditions and treatments are associated with constipation, and the symptoms associated with those other conditions are usually more obvious. When people say that constipation is their major symptom, the problem is usually IBS or idiopathic constipation.

Table 7.1 Causes of constipation

Cause	Comment
Lifestyle causes	
Inadequate fibre intake	Although this is often given as cause, most people with constipation do not in fact eat less fibre than those without it
Inadequate food	Constipation **always** follows starvation
Suppressing or ignoring the urge to defecate	This is possibly the most common cause
Immobility	Lack of movement is a common cause of constipation in those who are elderly and ill. Exercise increases bowel activity
Gastrointestinal causes	
Irritable bowel syndrome (IBS)	About a third of patients with IBS have mainly constipation (IBS-C), and IBS is one of the most frequent causes of constipation
Poor function and lack of co-ordination of the pelvic floor muscles. The doctor might call this pelvic floor dyssynergia or anismus	Defecation involves several muscle groups that need to contract and relax in the correct pattern. For example, the anal muscles must relax as the rectum contracts to push the stool out. If this does not happen, there is a feeling of blockage
Rectocoele	This is a bulging of the front wall of the rectum into the back wall of the vagina. It may mean that the force of defecation is directed towards the vagina rather than down towards the anus

Table 7.1 Causes of constipation *continued*

Cause	Comment
Medications	
Opiate-based analgesics such as codeine, dihydrocodeine, morphine, diamorphine and others	Constipation is a common side effect of powerful painkillers that contain opiates
Antidepressants of the tricyclic type, including amitriptyline, imipramine and lofepramine	Constipation is a side effect of this class of antidepressant. Despite this, low-dose amitriptyline is often used to treat IBS that has pain as its main symptom
Iron tablets	Iron tablets can also cause diarrhoea
Hormonal and metabolic causes	
Hypothyroidism (an underactive thyroid)	It is routine practice to take blood tests for thyroid function in people who go to the doctor with constipation, although in my experience it is rarely a factor
Hypercalcaemia (a raised blood calcium level)	People with a very high calcium level are ill with a variety of symptoms, including nausea, vomiting, fatigue, thirst and passing a lot of urine. Constipation is usually present but tends to be the least of their problems. Blood calcium levels are routinely measured in blood tests that may be taken to diagnose other problems
Porphyria	This is a very rare disorder of haemoglobin production –although I have often tested for porphyria in people with otherwise unexplainable symptoms, I have never diagnosed it. It can show up with severe abdominal pain and constipation. The initial diagnosis is with a simple urine test

Table 7.1 Causes of constipation *continued*

Cause	Comment
Neurological disease	
Parkinson's disease	Constipation is very common due to a combination of factors, including side effects from the drug treatment, deterioration of the nerves supplying the gut, and lack of mobility
Multiple sclerosis and spinal cord damage	In these, there is a combination of nerve damage and reduced mobility
Psychological causes	
Depression	Constipation is a common problem, probably because of a combination of factors, including the disease itself, reduced activity, reduced food intake and side effects from drug treatment
Anorexia nervosa	People with anorexia are usually very physically active, but exercise does not make up for the lack of food intake in terms of preventing constipation. Constipation is an inevitable consequence of starvation

I don't like using the toilets at work. If I feel I want to go, I try to hold on until I get home. Am I doing myself any harm?

One of the functions of the large bowel is to hold the stool until it is convenient to pass it. Suppressing the 'call to stool' from time to time is quite natural. But doing so on a regular basis may significantly slow the bowel and make it harder to recognise the signs of needing to go to the toilet.

In a fascinating experiment, healthy subjects were asked to ignore their normal bowel habit and hold on for as long as possible. Their bowel habit, and the time it took for food to pass through their bowel, was carefully assessed before and after this. After just 3 days of 'holding on', half as many stools were passed, and the whole bowel slowed down to such an extent that the total time taken for food to pass through it doubled!

But I still don't want to use the toilet at work. Do you have any other suggestions?

The bowel is naturally more active in the morning. You may be able to train your bowel to open before you go to work. But this does mean having enough time for a relaxed breakfast. Filling the stomach with food increases muscle activity in the bowel through a mechanism called the gastrocolic reflex. This will encourage the call to stool by increasing the strength of muscular contractions in the rectum and help with defecation. While your bowel is getting used to the new pattern, it may help to take a laxative before going to bed.

Are some people's bowels simply too slow?

Yes, it's called slow-transit constipation. We can measure the time it takes for food to pass through the gut by tracking the passage of small, solid, pill-sized balls along it. These balls are made of inert (unreactive) materials that show up on X-rays and are not digested in the gut. The average time it takes for something to travel the whole length of the gut is 50 hours. In over 95% of healthy people, the time is less than 70 hours. But in some constipated individuals, this time is prolonged by several days, and in severe cases by several weeks. It is a particular problem in young women, in whom the constipation is often associated with a lot of bloating and pain. People who have this 'slow-transit constipation' often say that they rarely feel a message to go to the toilet.

There are many reasons why people ignore the body's message that they need to go – no time to go to the toilet, no convenient toilet, too busy to hear the call to stool, or a painful or sore anus. Whatever the reason, it seems that the bowel slows down within a surprisingly short time. Moreover, the longer the stool remains within the bowel, the harder it will get as more water is absorbed from it. As a result, there is constipation, and in some people this will become an ongoing problem.

Why do I get constipated when I go on holiday?

This is a common problem. People often attribute it to a change in diet or a lack of fluid, but there are more likely explanations. It is usually just not convenient to listen to the call to stool in the rushed preparations before a holiday – and even less so while travelling. There is nothing wrong with occasionally ignoring or suppressing the urge to defecate, but you have to accept that the longer the stool remains in the bowel, the more water will be absorbed from it and the harder it will get. Stress, too, may slow the bowel down, even when the stress itself is part of the fun.

If I'm getting stressed, then, how will this affect my bowel?

In simple terms, the bowel is regulated by two sets of nerves: the sympathetic system and the parasympathetic system. The parasympathetic system tends to increase the secretion of digestive juices and speeds up the action of the bowel. The sympathetic system slows the bowel down. The sympathetic system has evolved to help us cope with periods of intense physical and mental stress. It diverts blood flow towards the brain and muscles and away from the gut and the kidneys. This is to help the 'fight or flight' response, maximising muscle strength and mental agility while temporarily lessening the function of other organs. In simple terms, you don't want to defecate while you are being chased by a lion. It's when the stress continues that constipation can become a problem.

I have depression as well as IBS. The antidepressants have really helped but they make me very constipated. I don't want to stop them. What can I do?

The constipating effect of some antidepressant drugs is due to an effect on the nerves supplying the bowel. The nerves that stimulate bowel activity (the parasympathetic system) communicate with the bowel by secreting a chemical called acetylcholine. This binds to specific receptors on the bowel cells that are called cholinergic receptors. Many drugs work by blocking cholinergic receptors – so they are said to have 'anticholinergic properties'. Some antidepressants work by blocking cholinergic receptors within the brain, and it is inevitable that they will have an effect on the rest of the body too, for example slowing the bowel. Although the constipation may be helped by more fibre and exercise, laxatives may be necessary.

I've been told I have a rectocoele. What is that?

The rectum lies directly behind the vagina. It is separated from the vagina by a thick, fibrous membrane that may weaken with age or if there has been any vaginal damage while giving birth. This means that when the pressure within the rectum increases to push the stool out during defecation, the front wall of the rectum may herniate (protrude through) this membrane, pushing into the back of the vagina. Defecation becomes difficult because the force becomes directed towards the back of the vagina rather than down towards the anus.

Sometimes a woman will report that defecation begins normally but never feels complete – the stool seems to get 'stuck' on the way out, and no amount of straining seems to shift it. Women develop manoeuvres to help, the most successful of which involves placing two fingers in the vagina to support its back wall. Treatment involves softening the stool with fibre and laxatives. You must avoid straining as this only worsens the condition. Occasionally, an operation may be necessary to repair it.

How do I know if I have just constipation, or whether it's IBS and constipation?

There is no clear-cut distinction but more of a continuum of symptoms. Some people just get constipated, and are completely better once their constipation has been relieved. Others have a more complicated problem with pain and bloating that persist even when their bowel is empty. The latter have IBS.

About a third of people with IBS tend to be constipated (denoted as IBS-C), a third tend to suffer from diarrhoea (called IBS-D), and a third suffer from both constipation and diarrhoea, with a mixed or alternating bowel habit described as IBS-A (or IBS-M). But some people are constipated without any other symptoms that suggest IBS. Table 7.2 is adapted from the criteria developed by an international group of experts to provide a standard way of identifying patients for clinical trials. These are known as the Rome criteria and are now also used in clinical practice.

According to these criteria, the most important difference between IBS-C and constipation is the amount of pain and abdominal discomfort in IBS. In practice, however, I do not find this distinction useful as most constipated people will be uncomfortable, and most of those with IBS-C will be more comfortable once their constipation has been relieved. Symptoms left over after relieving constipation that are not attributable to other conditions tend to be ascribed to IBS.

FIBRE AND CONSTIPATION

What is dietary fibre?

Dietary fibre is indigestible plant carbohydrate (mainly substances called cellulose, pectins and lignins from the plant's cell wall). It passes through the small bowel without being digested and into the large bowel, where bacteria partially metabolise it into gas, fluid and substances called short-chain fatty acids. These short-chain fatty

Table 7.2 The diagnostic criteria for irritable bowel syndrome (IBS) and constipation based on the Rome III conference published in 2006

Feature of IBS	Features of constipation
Recurrent abdominal discomfort or pain for at least 3 days per month in the last 3 months associated with two or more of the following: ■ Improvement with defecation ■ An onset of pain associated with a change in frequency of the stool ■ An onset of pain associated with a change in form (appearance) of the stool	The stools are not loose except with the use of laxatives, and there are insufficient criteria for IBS The person needs to have had symptoms for at least 6 months, and two of the following for the last 3 months: ■ Straining for more than 25% of the time ■ Lumpy or hard stools at more than 25% of defecations ■ A feeling of obstruction or blockage in the anus or rectum on more than 25% of defecations ■ Manual manoeuvres to help used on more than 25% of defecations ■ Fewer than three defecations a week

Other symptoms that, taken together, support the diagnosis of IBS include:

■ An abnormal frequency of passing stools (more than three a day or fewer than three a week)

■ An abnormal form of the stool (hard/lumpy or loose/watery) (see Figure 7.1)

■ An abnormal passage of the stool

■ Mucus (slime) being passed

■ Bloating or a feeling of abdominal distension

acids are absorbed by the large bowel and are an important nutrient for the bowel. Most of the rest of the fibre passes through the bowel in the stool, along with water and gas trapped in it and bacteria living on it. Fibre therefore produces a softer, wetter, bulkier stool that is easier to pass.

What is the difference between soluble and insoluble fibre?

There are two major types of fibre – soluble and insoluble (Table 7.3). Soluble fibre is broken down by bacteria in the colon to produce energy and gas, and bulky stools. This fibre forms a gel-like substance that can bind to other substances in the gut. It also has the extra benefits of lowering cholesterol levels and slowing down the entry of glucose into the blood, thereby improving blood sugar control. Insoluble fibre is less easily broken down by bacteria in the colon but holds water very effectively (up to 15 times its weight in water), which contributes to an increase in stool weight. It is this fibre that is often referred to as 'nature's broom' in that, by passing right through the gut, with extra water, it helps to clear the bowel out.

Plant foods contain a combination of both types of fibre, but some plants contain more of one type than the other.

Table 7.3 Sources of dietary fibre

Mainly soluble fibre	Mainly insoluble fibre
Fruit	The skin and pips of fruit and vegetables
Vegetables	Wholegrain cereals (wheat, rye, rice)
Pulses (peas, beans)	Nuts
Oats	
Barley	
Seeds	

Table 7.4 Results from two studies on dietary fibre

Diagnosis	Number of people studied	Fibre intake (g/day)	Fluid intake (litres/day)
People with slow bowels, defined by medical tests	64	14.7	1.2
People with normal bowels, defined by medical tests	64	15	1.2
People who say they are constipated	62	18.3	2.1
People who say they have a normal bowel habit	100	18.1	2.0

Am I eating too little fibre?

Surprisingly, most studies that have compared diet between people with and without constipation have found no difference in the amount of dietary fibre that they eat or the amount of fluid that they drink. Table 7.4 shows the results from two studies, although many more have been done. One explanation for these results is to say that most of us actually do not eat enough fibre, but only some of us are afflicted by constipation. In other words, fibre intake is only one factor.

So how much fibre should I have?

The usual recommendation is 30 g a day, but this is not easy to achieve! Table 7.5 shows the fibre content of some common foods.

The fibre content is given in the nutrition information that now comes with foodstuffs, and a full list can also be obtained from the US Department of Agriculture, Agricultural Research Service (see the Appendix).

Table 7.5 Fibre content of common foods

Food	Amount of fibre
Apple (with skin)	3.7 g
Orange	3 g
Banana	2.8 g
Wholemeal bread (1 slice)	2 g
Ryvita (1 slice)	1.9 g
Bowl of bran	10 g
Bowl of muesli	6 g
Bowl of cornflakes	1 g
Baked beans (small can)	7.4 g
Lettuce (1 leaf)	0.1 g
Lettuce (1 iceberg)	6.5 g
Tomato	1.5 g
Cucumber (large)	1.5 g
Pepper (1 sweet red, raw)	2.4 g
Grapes (10 grapes)	0.4 g
Nuts (24 almonds)	3.3 g
Potato (boiled in skin)	2.4 g
Oat bran (cooked, 1 cup)	5.7 g

If you want to use fibre to help your constipation, it is usually best to start with small additions of up to 10 g a day. Sachets of supplementary fibre usually contain 3.5–5 g of fibre.

But if I eat more fibre, will it help my constipation?

Eating more dietary fibre is the most common first recommendation made by healthcare professionals if someone with constipation comes to see them. Indeed, studies comparing psyllium (*Ispaghula* husk) or bran with a dummy treatment (placebo) have shown that the frequency and bulk of the stools increases with the fibre.

Although in my experience as a hospital specialist, fewer than 25% of constipated people are helped by an increase in dietary fibre, the limited success of fibre seen by specialists probably occurs because the people referred to them have the worst constipation. Those with less severe symptoms successfully treat themselves or are managed by their family doctor.

I tried taking more fibre, but it just made me more bloated without helping my bowel at all. Why is that?

The usual advice is to keep taking the extra fibre. The fibre may take several days to pass through your large bowel, and it takes time for the extra water that it holds in your bowel to have an effect. So until your bowel empties, it is probably inevitable that the extra bulk, and the wind generated as the bacteria digest some of the fibre, will make you feel more bloated. The excess bloating may well settle down as your bowel adjusts over a few weeks.

For some people, such as myself, life is too short to try this approach! The easiest way to relieve the constipation is with a laxative that stimulates the bowel to move. You can then use extra fibre to stop the problem coming back.

LAXATIVES

What are the different types of laxative that I could buy at a pharmacy?

Laxatives can be roughly divided into several groups; these are called bulk-forming, osmotic, emollient (also called faecal softeners) and stimulant (Table 7.6).

Bulk-forming laxatives

Bulk-forming laxatives are fibre. Like dietary fibre, they work by providing a surface area and nutrients for bacteria to grow and multiply, as well as by drawing water into the bowel. To help this, and to prevent the fibre congealing into a solid mass, you should drink plenty of fluid. The stool will then become bulkier and softer. Fibre does not directly stimulate the muscles of the bowel. It is usually said that the increased bulk of the stool stimulates the muscles of the bowel wall to push the stool out more quickly and that the increased softness of the stool helps this. But although most studies confirm that fibre increases stool bulk and relieves constipation, the time taken for food to pass through the bowel is not affected.

Because the fibre is metabolised by bacteria to make gas, bloating and flatulence are frequent side effects. Taking a bulking agent into an already full bowel usually leads to discomfort, at least to start with. Hence once you decide to treat your constipation with extra fibre, it is essential to persevere for at least a week if not longer.

Osmotic laxatives

Osmosis is the process by which water distributes itself so that the concentration of molecules dissolved within the water is equal between different parts of the body – balancing the concentrations out between these different parts. If we take in substances that are soluble in water but cannot be absorbed from the gut, we can draw water into the bowel from the body and keep it there.

The most commonly used osmotic laxative is a sugar called lactulose, which cannot be digested. It comes as a sweet-tasting syrup. Like sugar, it can absorb a great deal of water. But unlike ordinary sugar, it cannot be digested or absorbed, so it passes out unchanged in the stool. By holding a lot of water within the stool, lactulose softens the stool, and in large doses it can cause diarrhoea. Unfortunately, some bacteria within the bowel can metabolise lactulose to produce gas. Thus, wind and bloating are a common side effect. For most people lactulose is a safe, gentle but relatively weak laxative.

Magnesium is poorly absorbed from the gut, so magnesium salts also act as osmotic laxatives. When magnesium is combined with hydroxide as an alkali – to form magnesium hydroxide (Cream of Magnesia) – it is also a useful antacid. Magnesium can be a potent laxative in some people, such that some people who take magnesium supplements will complain of diarrhoea. Magnesium is also sometimes included in so-called 'natural' bowel cleansers or detoxifying products.

More recently, osmotic laxatives based on polyethylene glycols have been introduced. Polyethelene glycols are inert (unreactive), water-soluble compounds formed from ethylene oxide; they are a bit like polythene but soluble in water. They have a very high osmotic activity, meaning that they hold very large quantities of water. In addition, neither the human gut nor the bacteria in it digest them, and they pass right through the gut unchanged. They are more effective than other osmotic laxatives, with less bloating and wind as side effects. As well as being used as laxatives, they are also used as bowel-cleansing agents when the bowel needs to be cleaned out before surgery or tests such as colonoscopy.

Emollient laxatives

Emollient laxatives, also called faecal softeners, consist of mineral oil and docusate salts. Mineral oil can be given by mouth (orally) or by enema; it penetrates and softens the stool. The oldest of these laxatives is liquid paraffin. Although it was once frequently used both orally and as an enema, it is now rarely recommended, for a variety of reasons. It can interfere with vitamin absorption if taken regularly, and it can also be absorbed from the gut and deposited in the liver and spleen. Moreover, leakage of paraffin from the anus can irritate the skin. In previous times, when debilitated patients were encouraged to take liquid paraffin before bed, vomiting and aspiration in bed led to an unpleasant type of pneumonia.

An enema containing arachis (peanut) oil is still occasionally used to soften compressed and hardened stool in the lower bowel. This occasionally occurs in people with prolonged severe constipation, especially if they have been immobile. The bowel may be almost blocked by stool (sometimes called faecal impaction) allowing only water and wind to pass (sometimes called overflow diarrhoea).

Docusate and Dioctyl sodium preparations are sometimes classed as faecal softeners and sometimes as stimulant laxatives. They act mainly to reduce the surface tension of the stool, which allows a greater mixing of water and fat. They may also stimulate the bowel wall to secrete more fluid. Although they are still sold as laxatives, studies comparing them with an inactive treatment (a placebo) have failed to show any change in the water content of the stools, in stool weight, in frequency of defecation or in how long it takes the gut contents to go through the colon after docusates have been taken in the recommended doses, and it is unclear whether they do anything at all. They may, however, be worth trying if you want something very gentle.

Stimulant laxatives

Stimulant laxatives act predominantly by increasing muscle contractions in the bowel wall so that stool is passed more effectively. Castor oil has been known as a stimulant laxative since ancient times. It has an unpleasant taste and makes people sick, as well as leading to severe cramping pains, so very few people like taking it. Surprisingly, it may find a new role in stimulating labour at the end of pregnancy.

The anthraquinones are compounds produced by several different plants, including senna, casacara, frangula and rhubarb. They are metabolised by the bacteria in the large bowel to produce compounds that increase the secretion of water into the bowel and stimulate muscle activity in the bowel wall. A large variety are available at pharmacies without prescription. Like most herbal remedies, the preparations are unrefined and contain mixtures of various chemicals. It is therefore difficult to advise on a dose, but they are generally considered to be safe and effective. They usually work 8–12 hours after dosing so are commonly taken in the evening or before bed to promote the natural increase in bowel activity that occurs in the morning.

Bisacodyl is taken as a tablet and is available over the counter. It has to be converted to an active compound by bacteria in the large bowel and stimulates defecation 6–8 hours after being taken. The usual dose is 5–10 mg before bed, but the dose can be increased to 20 mg. Bisacodyl suppositories work much more quickly: within 15–30 minutes.

Sodium picosulphate is similar to bisacodyl and is also available as over-the-counter tablets. It is better known to generations of doctors, nurses and patients as the bowel-cleansing agent Picolax, in which it is combined with a magnesium salt (magnesium citrate) to produce a very powerful stimulant laxative.

So which laxative should I use?

This is very much a matter of trial and error. There is a lot of subjective opinion but very little experimental evidence of which laxative works best for different problems. Table 7.7 below gives some guidance, but I would encourage you to experiment for yourself.

Table 7.6 The different types of laxative available

Laxative	Common trade names (available without prescription)	Onset of action	Comments
Bulk-forming laxatives			Fibre preparations available over the counter
Ispaghula husk (psyllium)	Regulan, Fybogel, Metamucil (USA)	12–72 hours, but be prepared to give it longer	This is usually available as granules. It increases bloating, at least initially. Drink plenty of water
Sterculia	Normacol, Normacol plus	12–72 hours	This is a gum obtained from *Sterculia* plants
Methylcellulose	Celevac, Citrucel (USA)	12–72 hours	This is a synthetic soluble fibre, designed to produce less bacterial breakdown so less wind. It is available as tablets or a liquid
Osmotic laxatives			Hold water within the bowel
Lactulose	Duphalac, Lactugal, Regulose	Usually 0.5–3 hours, but can take as long as 24–48 hours	This comes as a sweet-tasting syrup. It can be diluted with water, fruit juice or milk, or taken in a food. It often causes bloating and wind. Lactulose is a relatively weak laxative

Magnesium hydroxide	Milk of Magnesia, Cream of Magnesia	0.5–3 hours	This is available as a liquid suspension. It can be potent and rapidly acting. Take plenty of fluids. It is to be avoided in renal failure
Magnesium sulphate	Epsom salts, Andrews Liver Salts or Original Andrews Salts	0.4–3 hours	This is more potent than magnesium hydroxide. It can cause severe bloating and sudden diarrhoea. Andrews Salts also contain sodium bicarbonate and citric acid so work as an antacid too
Polyethylene glycols	Movicol, Idrolax	1–2 hours but can be much longer in some people	This comes as a sachet of powder that is taken with water. It is probably as effective and more palatable than magnesium hydroxide
Emollient laxatives			Soften the stool
Liquid paraffin	Liquid paraffin oral emulsion	6–8 hours	This softens the stool and lubricates the intestine, but anal leakage of paraffin can be irritating
Arachis oil	Fletchers' Arachis Oil Retention Enema	5–15 minutes	This softens hard stool in the lower bowel. It come only as an enema. Do not use it if you are allergic to nuts
Docusate sodium	Dioctyl, Docusol, Norglass Micro-enema	12–72 hours when taken orally. A few minutes to 15 minutes as an enema	This has some bowel-stimulating activity as well as softening the stool. It is relatively mild

Table 7.6 The different types of laxative available *continued*

Laxative	Common trade names (available without prescription)	Onset of action	Comments
Stimulant laxatives			Stimulate muscular contraction in the bowel, which can be painful
Senna	Senokot, Manevac, Ex-lax Senna	8–12 hours	This is available as tablets, granules or a syrup
Bisacodyl	Dulco-lax (bisacodyl)	6–10 hours when taken orally; 15–30 minutes as a suppository	This comes as tablets or suppositories. It is probably more reliable than senna
Sodium picosulphate	Dulco-lax (sodium picosulphate), Laxoberal	6–10 hours	This is a potent stimulant laxative available as an elixir or tablets

Table 7.7 Guidance on which laxative to try first

Problem	Suggested laxative to try first
Large, hard, difficult-to-pass stools	A softening laxative such as lactulose or docusate
Separate small hard or soft lumps, sometimes difficult to pass	More fibre, or a bulk-forming laxative such as *Ispaghula*
Infrequent bowel movements, with bloating and discomfort	A stimulant laxative such as senna or bisacodyl
A feeling of fullness in the rectum, or a feeling of incomplete emptying	A glycerine or bisacodyl suppository, or both together

Are there any new types of medicine for constipation, or are the ones you've mentioned above the ones I should try?

Tegaserod is a new drug treatment for severe constipation and IBS that has constipation as its main feature (see Chapter 4). It is not yet licensed in the UK but hopefully will be soon.

What about enemas and suppositories?

You can buy laxatives to administer yourself directly into your rectum in the form of suppositories or enemas; they act in a similar way to the equivalent medicines taken by mouth. They usually work within 1 hour, and often within 15 minutes. Glycerine suppositories draw water into the rectum from the bowel wall. In this way, they soften the stool and, by increasing the volume within the rectum, can stimulate the passage of the stool. Bisacodyl suppositories can directly stimulate a bowel action, and a combination of a bisacodyl suppository with a glycerine suppository is sometimes helpful.

Enemas are more effective than suppositories but are more difficult to administer yourself. Phosphate enemas are often used in hospitals and can be used at home. They draw a large amount of water from the bowel wall into the gut. The resulting rapid distension of the lower bowel usually gives a very effective bowel motion.

I used to be very comfortable taking Ex-lax, but it's now no longer available. Why is that?

Ex-lax was popular on both sides of the Atlantic. It contained phenolphthalein, which was until recently the main component in numerous over-the-counter laxatives. As well as stimulating the large bowel, it reduced the absorption of fluid from the small bowel so that more water was delivered to the large bowel, which in turn gave softer stools. However, after a 2-year study showed that rats and mice fed 50–100 times the human dose of phenolphthalein developed various tumours, the US Food and Drug Administration reclassified phenolphthalein as 'not generally recognised as safe and effective'. Although the only data on laxative use and human cancers indicate that laxatives do not increase the risk of large bowel and other cancers, phenolphthalein-containing laxatives were voluntarily withdrawn and largely replaced with senna-containing compounds (Ex-lax Senna).

So do they actually know whether laxatives can cause cancer?

Cancer of the large bowel is the second most common cancer in people, so a great deal of research has been done on it. Although laxatives containing phenolphthalein were withdrawn due to fears of a cancer risk in animals (see the previous question), animal studies using currently available laxatives show no increased risk of cancer. Moreover, in the many studies of cancer of the bowel in humans, no association with laxative use, either past or present, has been shown.

I'm worried about laxatives damaging my bowel in some other way, though. Could this happen?

Laxatives are safe to use. The belief that they can damage the bowel when taken for prolonged periods is a myth.

But I have been told by several doctors and nurses to only use laxatives for a short period. Why do they think that there is a long-term problem with laxatives?

There is a widespread belief among healthcare professionals and lay people that stimulant laxatives used for any significant stretch of time can lead to permanent damage to the nerves and muscles of the bowel wall. The result is a bowel that is even slower than before, so the person ends up dependent on laxatives to keep it going. Stimulant laxatives are therefore traditionally recommended only for short-term use, meaning a few days to a few weeks. However, the idea that they can damage the bowel is so prevalent that many individuals and their doctors will not consider using these compounds even for severe constipation, relying instead on the less effective fibre preparations. Even osmotic laxatives, which have never been suggested to have a detrimental effect on long-term health, have been tarred with the same brush.

There are several reasons why people believe that stimulant laxatives can damage the bowel. A study published in 1968 looked at large bowels surgically removed in an attempt to relieve severe constipation. These showed damage to the nerves supplying the bowel (the enteric nerves) and wasting of the muscle in the bowel wall. Further studies in later years confirmed an association between long-term severe constipation, laxative use and enteric nerve damage. But most of the patients studied had used laxatives for more than 10 years in daily doses that exceeded the recommended daily dose by a factor of 18! Moreover, it is far from clear whether the damage seen was due to laxatives no longer in current use, to taking laxatives still available, to excessive doses or to a disease process of the large bowel itself that, by causing the constipation in the first place, meant that the laxatives were taken to try and cure it. Indeed, damage to the enteric nerves is seen in conditions that specifically affect the bowel, such as inflammatory bowel disease, and in diseases that affect nerve function generally, such as diabetes.

More recently, it has been shown that individuals with severely slow bowels (what is called colonic inertia) have fewer nerve cells in their bowel wall. The implication is that this is the initial problem, part of the disease itself, and not a consequence of laxative use. Furthermore, a study that compared the structure of nerves in the bowel wall between constipated people taking stimulant laxatives and constipated people not taking laxatives showed no significant difference.

In summary, modern research does not support the idea that laxatives induce bowel damage. It is therefore unlikely that stimulant laxatives used regularly in the recommended doses will harm the bowel.

I recently had a colonoscopy. They looked around my bowel with a camera, took samples and told me that I had 'melanosis coli' – damage to the bowel wall caused by laxatives. What is this?

Melanosis coli is an easily seen brown pigmentation of the bowel wall. It may occur within months if you regularly use anthraquinone laxatives such as senna or rhubarb. It can last for months after stopping laxative use.

Each cell in the lining of the bowel lives for about 6 days before it dies and is replaced. Its debris is taken up by scavenger cells called macrophages. Anthraquinone laxatives stain this debris, so when it is taken up by macrophages, it gives the bowel wall a brown discolouration. This is of no clinical significance. In fact, it makes it easier to spot other, more important problems if you are having a colonoscopy.

Will I become dependent on laxatives once I start using them?

Most people use laxatives intermittently, just when they feel constipated. This may be every few days, every week or just occasionally. Some people do have to use them regularly to avoid constipation. There is nothing wrong with this. If you stop using them, the worst that can happen is constipation, and it will be no worse than the constipation you had before you started.

If I continue to use laxatives, will they become less effective? Will I need to continually increase the dose of laxative that I use?

It has been said that, after months or years of regular use, the bowel's response to laxatives will diminish, so larger and larger doses will be needed to give the same effect. This is said to be a particular problem with stimulant laxatives, which are recommended for short-term use only. Indeed, in one small study, two-thirds of patients currently using sodium picosulphate (a strong stimulant laxative) claimed to have increased their dose over 10–20 years of use. We don't know whether this was because the laxative became less effective or because their constipation got worse with time.

In animal studies, senna-type laxatives and bisacodyl (a stimulant laxative) were given to rats and mice in large doses for prolonged periods without any signs of loss of effect. Moreover, in a study looking at people with spinal cord injuries who required bisacodyl (a stimulant laxative), no loss of effect was seen over periods ranging from 2 to 34 years.

In summary, although some patients with severe constipation undoubtedly do need to increase their use of laxatives over time, this is more likely to reflect worsening constipation. In most people regularly using standard doses of laxatives, no tolerance develops, and the laxative remains effective. So you are highly unlikely to become dependent on your laxative.

I've been told that, if I use laxatives, I could lose too much potassium from my body.

In clinical practice, it is not unusual to see patients with a low blood potassium level (called hypokalaemia) which makes them feel tired and weak. In people with gastroenteritis, for example, large amounts of potassium may be lost in the watery stool, with little food or drink being taken to replace it. A similar situation may arise in people who abuse laxatives to lose weight. But in studies that followed people taking senna for over 1 year, there was no disturbance in the levels of potassium or of other minerals in the blood.

Do laxatives have a role in weight loss?

Laxatives are sometimes taken in doses big enough to cause diarrhoea to 'help' with weight loss – presumably in the belief that diarrhoea will prevent food that has been eaten from being absorbed. But this belief is entirely false. Laxatives predominantly affect the large bowel, whereas nutrients are absorbed in the small bowel. All that enters the large bowel is water and waste. The weight loss brought about by laxative-induced diarrhoea is due to dehydration. There is no loss of fat.

OVERFLOW CONSTIPATION AND DIARRHOEA

I've suffered from diarrhoea for a long time. Some days, I would just gush out a small piece of stool followed by lots of water. This could happen several times a day. Oddly, on other days, I wouldn't need to go at all. Eventually, I was seen at a hospital clinic. They said I was constipated and told me to take laxatives! How can this be?

This is called overflow constipation. I see it regularly, even in fit and active young people. Figure 7.3 is an X-ray of an active,

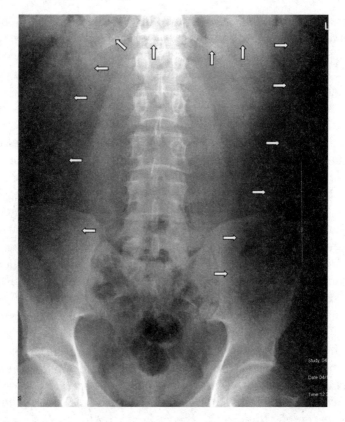

Figure 7.3 An X-ray of the abdomen from a man with constipation.

42-year-old man who was suffering from intermittent diarrhoea and bloating. The arrows are pointing to his colon, which is full of stool all the way round; it looks like fluffy shadows. If the bowel were not full of stool, it would be outlined only by the air within it, which looks black on the X-ray.

There is not necessarily anything wrong with this situation – after all, it's the function of the colon to hold stool, and there's no problem if the bowel and its owner are comfortable. But when the colon holds more stool than it's happy with, it may try to excrete the stool by secreting more water and mucus. If the stool is hard and impacted (gets stuck) within the bowel, the water may bypass the stool and come out as just a very watery stool with perhaps some pieces of solid stool within it. So the person thinks that he or she has diarrhoea.

The doctor may find several clues to the right diagnosis. First, the diarrhoea is intermittent, with days of no bowel activity at all, and the abdomen may appear full or distended. If a rectal examination is performed, there may be hard stool within the rectum. The diagnosis can be confirmed by a simple abdominal X-ray like the one in Figure 7.3. Without the X-ray, it can be very difficult to explain to a young man complaining of diarrhoea that he is actually constipated!

When this gentleman had his X-ray explained to him, he was able to understand his symptoms of frequent bowel motions and spasms, as the bowel tried to empty itself. The treatment he was offered also made sense to him. I would like to say that I always spot this diagnosis straight away, but in fact I believe I more often make it in retrospect.

I have always had an irregular bowel habit – sometimes constipated, sometimes loose. More recently, my bowel habit's changed and I went to see my doctor about constant diarrhoea. Eventually, I had a colonoscopy. They told me that my bowel was completely normal. I received no treatment, but for the first week or two after the colonoscopy my bowel habit was better than it had ever been. Now it's all starting up again – sometimes constipation, sometimes diarrhoea. What can I do?

There are a number of possible explanations for why you felt so much better after the colonoscopy. First, the reassurance of knowing that there is nothing seriously amiss can greatly help symptoms. This is true even in people who are not overtly anxious. More intriguing is the possibility that your symptoms are due to overflow constipation, so that the periods of diarrhoea represent an attempt by your bowel to clear itself. The day before the colonoscopy, you would have taken large doses of powerful laxatives to clear your bowel of stool. This is usually the worst part of the procedure, but in your case, by clearing the constipation, it might have been therapeutic! You can test this hypothesis by taking laxatives. You will not need to be as drastic with the laxatives as you were before the colonoscopy, and standard doses of senna or bisacodyl for a few days may do.

PROBLEMS AND SOLUTIONS

I'm 23 and I get pain low down on the left side of my abdomen. It's a cramping pain that comes and goes, and I get it several times a week. If I can get my bowels open really well, it gets much better, but I usually pass small hard stools with a lot of effort. Am I constipated, or is this something more serious?

It sounds very much like constipation. The bowel in the left lower corner of the abdomen where you get your pain is called the sigmoid colon (see Figure 1.1). Its function is to hold the stool until you are ready to expel it. The pain you describe is a spasmodic contraction of the sigmoid colon as it tries to expel the hard stool.

The usual advice is to drink plenty of water, eat more fibre and take more exercise. This will work in many cases, but it may take time and may initially make you a little worse as well as bloated. Another strategy is to take a stimulant laxative like senna or bisacodyl before bed and you will probably open your bowel well in the morning. You may need to do this for several days to get it clear enough, passing soft stools and feeling that your bowel has emptied. It may then be possible to avoid any more constipation by eating a little more fibre and taking more exercise. However, there is nothing wrong with using stimulant laxatives every so often.

I tried using senna but it gave me the same spasm-like pain in the lower left corner of my abdomen that was bothering me in the first place!

Cramping pains or spasms are a side effect of stimulant laxatives. You can think of it in terms of the laxative stimulating your bowel to contract around the hard stool. Once the stool has cleared, the pain will go.

You may prefer to try non-stimulant laxatives. A popular mild laxative is lactulose. This is a non-digestible sugar that softens the stool by drawing water into the bowel. Bacteria in the bowel are able to metabolise lactulose, producing gas, so bloating and wind are the main side effects. It is also sometimes not sufficiently strong enough. The laxatives based on polyethylene glycol (see a previous question) are also non-stimulating and are more effective, but they tend to be more expensive. They are available without prescription as Movicol or Idrolax. Older remedies, still popular, are magnesium salts such as Cream of Magnesia (magnesium hydroxide), Epsom salts (magnesium sulphate) and Andrews Liver Salts (magnesium sulphate, sodium bicarbonate and citric acid).

Does it do any harm to combine different kinds of laxative?

No, not at all. In fact, combinations may well work better. Fibre may be combined with a stimulant laxative; for example, Manevac is a combination of the fibre *Ispaghula* and the stimulant laxative senna. Stimulant laxatives often combine well with osmotic laxatives such as lactulose, polyethylene glycol or magnesium. It's worth trying different combinations to find what works for you.

I get a lot of pain in my abdomen. It's mostly low down on the right, but sometimes it's on the left, and sometimes the whole of the lower part of my abdomen aches with a kind of heavy, dragging feeling. I also get a lot of bloating, and sometimes I feel sick. My bowel habit has always been irregular, usually with small, pellet-like stools. I've had these symptoms for many years, and my GP has put them down to IBS. Recently I've noticed that if I open my bowels really well, the pain tends to ease. Could I be constipated?

The symptoms you describe are typical of IBS, and a third of people with IBS are also constipated (denoted as 'IBS-C'). If people open their bowels infrequently and produce hard stools, then yes, they are clearly constipated. Occasionally, however, people will pass stool on most days without actually clearing their bowel well enough. The bowel in IBS is more sensitive to being distended, be this with gas, liquid or solid stool, and pain that is improved by defecation is actually a part of the definition of IBS. It follows that some individuals with IBS will feel better if their bowels are emptied more thoroughly, especially if they are constipated.

By examining your abdomen, a doctor can sometimes tell if your bowel is full. Occasionally, I arrange an abdominal X-ray to see just how full a person's bowel really is. But it's often easier just to try some laxatives. Most people with your symptoms will also have been advised to increase the fibre content of their diet.

I did try sachets of Fybogel (Ispaghula husk). When I used two sachets a day, my stools did become softer and more formed, in larger pieces. I was going more regularly and I had less pain. It was the bloating I couldn't stand. I was promised that it would go, but it persisted and it's much worse with any other fibre preparation that I've tried. What can I do?

Unfortunately, bloating and wind are the consequence of taking more fibre. Sometimes it settles with time, but sometimes it doesn't. One solution is to use smaller quantities of fibre together with a laxative. Stimulant laxatives are simple to take but can cause spasm. Osmotic laxatives, especially polyethylene glycol, may be as effective without spasm. It is worth experimenting. There is a balance to be struck: more fibre will give better stools but more bloating; less fibre gives less wind, but the constipation may be worse. Trying fibre in combination with laxatives, either regularly or intermittently, may be more suitable.

I've had an irritable bowel for many years. The worst problem for me is the cramping, spasmy pain in my lower abdomen. I've tried all the antispasmodics available at the chemist and several that my doctor prescribed, but the only thing that helps is codeine. My problem with codeine, though, is that it constipates me. My stools become hard, I have to strain, and I generally feel even more bloated. My doctor suggested senna, but it just gives me more spasms. What do you suggest?

Codeine is an opioid-based analgesic (painkiller) but does cause a considerable slowing of the bowel. I would begin by making sure that the whole problem isn't just constipation that you are exacerbating with the codeine. Try to get a really good clear out with a laxative. That means taking enough laxative to pass a lot more stool than usual and making your stool much looser for a few days. Avoid taking codeine for those few days and see if you can weather the spasms over that time, or just take the antispasmodics. Try and use polyethylene glycol-based laxatives or other osmotic laxatives because stimulant laxatives such as senna can cause spasms and may continue to do so for 12 hours or more.

If you are much better after the clear out, or if your spasms are less severe and can be controlled by simple antispasmodics like peppermint oil, it's fine to repeat the laxative treatment whenever you need it.

But if your spasms persist despite clearing any constipation, the problem is how to continue using codeine without getting constipated. Taking more fibre in your diet will probably work, but you may find you have more bloating and wind. It might be better to introduce the extra fibre slowly, perhaps taking less than 5 g (about one sachet of fibre supplement or two fruits) each day in addition to your normal diet in the first week, and increasing the dose in the following weeks if necessary. Alternatively, small doses of an osmotic laxative taken routinely will keep the stool soft.

I eat a high-fibre diet with plenty of fluid, I exercise regularly, and I'm not taking any medication. But I'm always constipated. What am I doing wrong?

You're not doing anything wrong; life is just like that. I suggest that you take some laxatives and congratulate yourself on not having anything more serious and on looking after yourself well.

CONCLUSION

There are and always have been myths around constipation. Most doctors will now agree that a regular bowel habit is not essential for health and that a constipated bowel does not poison the body. But constipation is still a common problem both on its own and as part of IBS. Whichever is the case, relieving the constipation will usually help with bloating and pain as well as making defecation easier and more comfortable.

Most doctors and other healthcare professionals advise extra fibre and fluids as the first treatment for constipation. Contrary to the evidence that is available, many professionals advise against laxatives except as a last resort. Consequently, many people suffer for years before being given 'permission' by a doctor to use the simple treatments readily available at the chemist. If you suspect that constipation is part of your problem, it is worth trying some of the treatments described above. They are mostly available without prescription and are safe. Some people just try a fibre preparation and give up if it doesn't work or produces too much bloating. But if one laxative does nothing for you, or causes problems, try another of a different type. Don't be afraid of using potent stimulating laxatives to clear out your bowel.

SUMMARY

- A third of people with IBS will have constipation as their predominant problem.

- We are usually unable to determine a specific cause for the constipation.

- Constipation is rarely caused by serious bowel disorders.

- Some people just have a slow bowel.

- Exercise is important. As well as its other benefits, it keeps the bowel going.

- Stress usually slows the bowel.

- Eating too little fibre may cause or exacerbate constipation.

- Although in general people with constipation do not eat less fibre than people with a more usual bowel habit, eating more fibre may help and is the most commonly recommended first treatment.

- Fibre often makes the bloating of constipation worse, especially at first.

- Laxatives are effective and safe.

- The view that laxative use damages the bowel is a myth.

8 | Diarrhoea and faecal incontinence

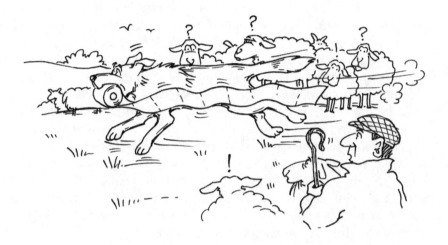

About one third of people with irritable bowel syndrome (IBS) have diarrhoea as one of their main problems. In many people, this can be controlled with simple measures, but in others the unpredictability of the bowel is a major problem. Unfortunately, some people are diagnosed as having diarrhoea-predominant IBS (IBS-D) when in fact they have another condition such as coeliac disease. This chapter will look at diarrhoea in IBS but will also describe other conditions that cause diarrhoea and can be mistaken for IBS.

Diarrhoea is the normal response of the bowel to infection or the presence of toxins. Increased muscle activity in the bowel wall, increased secretion of fluid into the gut and reduced absorption of the fluid all serve to help expel the infecting bacteria and toxins. Regardless of the cause, the symptoms usually feel the same – spasmodic abdominal pains accompanied by the need to rush to the toilet (urgency), where loose or watery stools are produced.

This process is usually self-limiting, ending within a few days or at most a few weeks. Problems arise if the process continues for some reason. For example, the infection giardiasis can persist in the small bowel for months or years. In coeliac disease, inflammation in the small bowel carries on because the immune system wrongly mounts a response to wheat. In inflammatory bowel disease (Crohn's disease and ulcerative colitis), the cause of the inflammation remains unknown but can be severe enough to be life-threatening. And in IBS too, low-grade inflammation, together with disordered control mechanisms, has been suggested as the cause of diarrhoea.

Bowel habit varies greatly between people, and an individual's bowel habit will also vary over time. In surveys, up to a quarter of people report passing a loose stool at some time during the previous month. The occasional loose stool is probably due to something that was eaten or drunk, or even to unaccustomed exercise. Diarrhoea that lasts a few days or weeks is likely to be due to infection with viruses or bacteria. It can be very unpleasant but will normally settle without treatment. People usually seek advice if the symptoms are intolerably severe or if they last for more than a few weeks. They may expect an instant answer from their doctor, but unfortunately it can be difficult to distinguish between the myriad of conditions that present with diarrhoea and abdominal pain.

> *I'm opening my bowels far more frequently than I used to, and with softer stools. My stools are formed, soft blobs, or smooth and sausage-like. Is that diarrhoea?*

Diarrhoea generally means watery stools, mushy stools or fluffy pieces with indistinct edges (see Figure 7.1 in Chapter 7). What you are describing is a change in your bowel habit to looser more frequent stools, but not amounting to diarrhoea. There may be many causes, such as a change in your diet, greater caffeine intake or your exercise regime, as discussed in the questions below, but if you are older than 50, you should see your doctor to consider the possibility of more serious problems.

Could it be cancer?

The idea that it could be cancer suggests itself to most people who suffer from diarrhoea at some time. Indeed, it also worries their doctors. We are right to be a little obsessed with cancer of the large bowel (colon cancer or colorectal cancer). It is fairly common, with an average lifetime risk of 1 in 25 (compared with a risk of breast cancer in women of 1 in 16, and of prostate cancer in men of 1 in 6). Cancer of the large bowel causes about 20 000 deaths in the UK and about 50 000 deaths in the USA each year. More importantly, it develops slowly over 5–10 years, and it is potentially curable. At present, only about half of the people diagnosed with colon cancer are cured. But if it can be diagnosed at an early stage, or even when it is just a polyp (a small mushroom-like growth, usually not yet malignant), the cure rate can be much higher.

A change in the bowel habit to looser, more frequent stools that lasts for more than a few weeks may represent the first sign of bowel cancer. People with this symptom, especially if they are over the age of 50 (bowel cancer is rare under this age), usually need to have their bowel investigated; this normally involves a colonoscopy or a barium enema (see Chapter 13 for an explanation of these tests). Excluding bowel cancer as the cause of the diarrhoea is undoubtedly the most important role for the doctor. Unfortunately, once we are sure that the symptoms are not due to cancer, it becomes all too easy to attribute them to an irritable bowel. This may be true in most cases, but in others relatively simple diagnoses are being missed, hidden by the relief that it isn't cancer. Part of the role of this chapter is to show how other conditions can masquerade as IBS.

A problem for people with IBS is knowing whether investigation is necessary at all. One of the key questions a doctor asks in order to determine whether it is necessary to investigate a person's bowel is 'Has your bowel habit changed?' But people with IBS often have such a disordered bowel habit that they cannot say if and when it has changed! Certainly, symptoms that have gone on for years are unlikely to be caused by cancer, but it is also possible that the symptoms of a 'new' cancer are being masked by those of a long-standing irritable bowel. Whether or not people with IBS will have a colonoscopy or a barium enema to look at their bowel will very much depend on how they describe their symptoms, on their age and on when they had their last test.

Another problem is the embarrassment some people feel in describing certain symptoms. They may complain of diarrhoea when what they actually suffer from is leakage of the faeces, anal soreness or even frank incontinence of their stool. In others, the loose stool may not be as much of a problem as having to rush to a toilet at unpredictable times. This is called urgency of stool and denotes a problem with the rectum. Other people have to rush to the toilet frequently but then pass very little; these people may in fact turn out to be constipated (see Chapter 7). So it is vital that symptoms are defined as accurately as possible if the right diagnosis is to be reached.

THE CAUSES OF DIARRHOEA

I've had diarrhoea for almost a month now. What could be causing it?

Diarrhoea that continues for more than a few weeks has many causes; the most common are shown in Table 8.1. In otherwise well people, IBS is the most likely cause.

I've had a change in my bowel habit over the past 2 months. I used to open my bowel once or twice a day with a formed stool, but now I go three or four times a day with a loose stool. I don't pass any blood or mucus, and I don't have to rush to the toilet. Apart from the loose stools, I'm a well 62-year-old man. What should I do?

You should see your doctor. He may find a simple explanation for the change in your bowel habit, such as a new medication or a

Table 8.1 Causes of persisting diarrhoea

Cause	Comment
Infections	
Giardiasis	This is infection of the small bowel with a tiny, single-celled organism. It is commonly acquired on holiday
Small bowel bacterial overgrowth	Occasionally, relatively harmless bacteria manage to proliferate in the normally sterile small bowel (see a later section in this chapter, and Chapter 3). They cause diarrhoea by impairing digestion and absorption. This is a common problem in those who are diabetic or elderly, and in people who have had surgery involving the small bowel
Inflammatory bowel disease	There is excessive activity of the immune system in the gut. Its cause is unknown
Ulcerative colitis	This affects only the large bowel. There is a need to rush quickly to the toilet (urgency of stool), usually with blood and mucus mixed in the stool
Crohn's disease	Abdominal pain and weight loss are common. Blood tests are often abnormal
Cancer of the bowel	The average lifetime risk of bowel cancer is 1 in 25. The most common symptoms are a change in the bowel habit to looser, more frequent stools, and anaemia. It is rare under the age of 50
Coeliac disease	This is an immune reaction to gluten, a constituent of wheat and barley. The immune system damages the lining of the small bowel. Food is therefore poorly digested and absorbed. Coeliac disease may affect up to 1 in 100 people and can show up at any age. There is a simple blood test to screen for coeliac disease

Table 8.1 Causes of persisting diarrhoea *continued*

Cause	Comment
Irritable bowel syndrome	Diarrhoea is common in this. However, it is not associated with weight loss or bleeding, and does not usually occur at night
Medications	
Metformin	Metformin is commonly used in diabetes
Antidepressants (the type known as selective serotonin reuptake inhibitors)	These include Prozac (fluoxetine), Cipramil (citalopram) and Seroxat (paroxetine)
Theophylline	This is a drug used in asthma
Laxatives	There are people who knowingly take laxatives yet complain of diarrhoea!
Food	
Lactose intolerance	Lactose is the sugar in dairy products. A proportion of adults lose the ability to digest this sugar, which then acts as a laxative
Fructose and sorbitol intolerance	Fructose is the main sugar in honey, many fruits and chocolate. In combination with glucose, it makes up sucrose, or table sugar. Sorbitol is used as a sweetener in ice cream, chewing gum, jam and diabetic foods. It is converted to fructose in the intestine. Some people have a lowered absorption of fructose, which then acts as a laxative
Caffeine	Caffeine stimulates and speeds up the bowel. It is present in cola drinks, coffee, tea and chocolate
Alcohol	Excess alcohol over a prolonged period frequently causes diarrhoea. It can take several weeks of abstinence for the bowel to recover
Dietary fibre	Whatever the cause of the diarrhoea, increasing the fibre intake will usually make it worse

change in your diet. If, after the change has been removed, your bowel returns to normal, all well and good. Otherwise, you need to be referred to the hospital to make sure that you don't have bowel cancer. This will usually involve an examination of your bowel with a flexible sigmoidoscopy and barium enema or a colonoscopy (Chapter 13 explains these medical investigations, which involve inserting a tube with a small camera on into the lower end of your bowel).

I recently had a colonoscopy to investigate the change in my bowel habit. They told me my bowel was completely normal, but I still have loose stools several times a day. What could it be, and what should I do?

People's bowel habit does change with life. We take it especially seriously in people over the age of 50 because a change in bowel habit to loose stools may represent the beginning of bowel cancer. It's possible that your current bowel habit is now the new 'norm' for you. If you are comfortable with this, nothing more needs to be done. However, it could be due to a number of other causes, some of which have simple solutions (see below). Some doctors, if they feel the risk of cancer is low, will actually look for these relatively simple causes of diarrhoea before embarking on a colonoscopy. If they were not considered prior to your colonoscopy, they should certainly be considered now.

LACTOSE INTOLERANCE

I've heard of people getting diarrhoea from milk and other dairy products. How does this happen?

Lactose is a natural sugar contained in dairy products (milk, butter, cheese and to a lesser extent yoghurt). To digest it, we need the enzyme lactase. An enzyme is a protein made by cells to help chemical reactions, and there are many enzymes attached to the inside wall of the small bowel to help digest our food. Lactase acts on the lactose in the food, transforming it into glucose, which can then be absorbed. Some people lose most of their lactase in adulthood – this can happen to as many as 15% of Caucasians and up to 100% of Asians. Lactase may also be lost temporarily for up to 6 months following an infection.

If this happens, the lactose remains undigested as it passes down the small bowel. As with other sugars, it avidly draws water onto itself, and it holds the water in the bowel. As a result, more water enters the large bowel, and the stool becomes softer or even loose. In some people, a glass of milk per day can be sufficient to cause diarrhoea. Bacteria in the large bowel do digest some of the lactose to produce gas, so lactose intolerance is often accompanied by wind and bloating as well as loose stools.

Why do some people get lactose intolerance?

Actually, we believe that lactose intolerance is the 'normal' adult human condition and that man became tolerant to lactose simply because of a genetic mutation that meant the lactase enzyme continued to be produced into adulthood across some of the species. Lactase activity is high during infancy, but in most mammals, including most humans, it declines after weaning.

If lactose intolerance is the 'norm' in human adults, how is it that many adults tolerate dairy products without problems?

Mutations in our genetic heritage often happen, but a mutation only becomes widespread if it offers some reproductive advantage to the individual possessing it. About 9000 years ago, humans began to domesticate cows, and milk became abundant for adults rather than just breast-feeding infants. Individuals who continued to produce the enzyme lactase were thus favoured as more of them were healthy and survived to have children, so the mutation became more prevalent through the process of natural selection. In some people, bacteria in the large bowel digest most of the lactose.

How can I find out if I've got lactose intolerance?

The simple way to find out if your symptoms are due to lactose intolerance is to avoid dairy products (milk, butter, cheese, yoghurt and milk chocolate). You should notice a dramatic improvement within a few days and certainly within a week. It is important to make sure that any improvement is not just a coincidence by then deliberately going back on dairy products to see if the symptoms recur. Even if you become convinced that your symptoms are due to lactose intolerance and you choose to avoid eating dairy products (see a later question about the effect of this on health), you should try to reintroduce them from time to time as the absence of lactase may just be temporary.

I have lactose intolerance but I sometimes just can't resist a cream cake and a bowl of ice cream! I pay for it afterwards with bloating and diarrhoea, but am I actually doing myself any harm?

The lactase is just acting as a laxative. It does you no harm at all. Enjoying the occasional cream cake will undoubtedly do you more good!

I have lactose intolerance. Is there anything I can do to reduce my symptoms?

Most people with lactose intolerance can tolerate small amounts of dairy products, for example still having milk in their coffee, and some dairy products are easier to tolerate than others. Hard cheese contains less lactose than soft cheese, and yoghurts are well tolerated because much of the lactose has already been fermented (broken up). Goats' milk or cheese contains about 10% less lactose than cows' milk, and soya milk has no lactose at all as it is of plant origin. Lactose-reduced cows' milk products are also available. Drops or capsules containing the lactase enzyme are available and reduce symptoms when they are taken with dairy products. Do try all of these as they may help.

If you continue to eat dairy products, the bacteria in your large bowel that can metabolise lactose will be favoured over the others. As a result, your ability to tolerate lactose will increase. Conversely, if you avoid lactose altogether, you will have fewer lactose-digesting bacteria and your ability to tolerate lactose will get worse. Finding the balance between eating dairy products and getting symptoms is a personal choice.

Will my lactose intolerance cause me any long-term harm?

Only if it means you don't get enough calcium in your diet – calcium is needed for healthy bones and teeth. Unfortunately, people who feel themselves to be lactose intolerant usually restrict their intake of dairy products but fail to make up their calcium intake. For example, a large survey from Finland, involving almost 12 000 middle-aged women, found that those with lactose intolerance consumed significantly less calcium (570 mg a day) than lactose-tolerant women (850 mg a day). Furthermore, the women who were lactose intolerant were more likely to require hormone-replacement therapy, or suffer a chronic health disorder or a bone fracture. There have also been other studies showing lower bone densities in people who are lactose intolerant.

It seems possible that people who experience symptoms following a generous serving of milk may avoid milk products in future despite the fact that smaller servings could be tolerated. Avoiding milk tends to make people more intolerant to it in the future because the bacteria in the large bowel will become less able to ferment the lactose efficiently. If avoiding dairy products becomes normal behaviour, bone density is likely to fall over a number of years, increasing the risk of osteoporosis and bone fractures.

If I decide to cut back on dairy products, where can I get more calcium from?

Only a limited choice of foods contain significant amounts of calcium – Table 8.2 shows some foods containing higher levels of calcium. The recommended daily intake of calcium for an adult (the RDA) is 800 mg. Supplement tablets don't cost too much and usually contain 300–500 mg of calcium.

The calcium content is sometimes given in the nutritional information that now comes with foodstuffs. A full list can also be obtained from the US Department of Agriculture, Agricultural Research Service (see the Appendix).

Table 8.2 Sources of calcium

Food	Calcium content (mg)
Plain yoghurt (small pot)	452
Rhubarb, frozen, cooked and with sugar (1 cup)	348
Atlantic sardine, canned in oil and then drained (small can, including the bones)	325
Milk, low-fat (1 cup)	290
Spinach, cooked, boiled, drained and served without salt (1 cup)	245
Beans, white with mature seeds, canned (1 cup)	191
Pink salmon, canned, including the liquid and bones (small can)	181
White long-grain rice, parboiled and enriched (1 cup, dry)	111
Soya milk (1 cup)	93

Is fructose intolerance anything like lactose intolerance?

Fructose is the main sugar found in honey, many fruits and chocolate, and in combination with glucose it makes sucrose or table sugar. Sorbitol in the diet is also converted to fructose in the intestine. Sorbitol is used as a sweetener in ice cream, chewing gum, jam and diabetic foods. It may also form the base of some medicinal preparations such as antacids and multivitamins.

Some people have diminished fructose absorption. So if they happen to take more fructose than they are used to, the extra fructose will fail to be absorbed and will pass on into the large bowel. Here it will hold water within the bowel, acting as a laxative.

Fructose intolerance is a cause of watery diarrhoea and bloating. Avoiding fructose should alleviate the symptoms within a few days. If you have fructose intolerance but prefer to put up with a little diarrhoea after eating fruit and chocolate, no harm will be done.

SMALL BOWEL BACTERIAL OVERGROWTH

I have heard of bacteria living in the stomach causing ulcers, and I have heard of 'good' bacteria living in the large bowel. Are there any bacteria in the small bowel?

The small bowel, where most of our digestion and absorption takes place, is normally almost sterile. It harbours few if any bacteria. By contrast, the large bowel is full of bacteria so that half the content of the usual stool is made up of bacterial cell bodies.

There are a number of mechanisms that keep the small bowel sterile. Acid in the stomach kills most of the bacteria that we ingest with our food. In addition, continuous rapid propulsion within the small bowel prevents the formation of stagnant pools of nutrients where bacteria can breed, and clears away any bacteria that have migrated up from the large bowel. There is also a valve between the small bowel and the large bowel that limits backflow.

But these mechanisms may fail, allowing bacteria to enter and pro-liferate within the small bowel. An excessive number of bacteria in the small bowel interfere with the digestion and absorption of food, caus-ing diarrhoea. There may also be bloating, wind and weight loss. This syndrome is called small bowel bacterial overgrowth. Surprisingly, the bacteria do not actually invade the body from the small bowel, so there are no symptoms of infection. People with small bowel bacterial overgrowth do not usually feel unwell and do not have a fever. They usually report having diarrhoea, which can be watery or fatty. Alternatively, they may just feel that they have an irritable bowel.

Who gets small bowel bacterial overgrowth?

Anyone can get this disorder, but some people are more likely to. Elderly people produce less acid to sterilise their food, their immune system may be weaker, and the propulsive movement of their small bowel may not be as co-ordinated. In those with diabetes, those who have had surgery on their small bowel and those who have nerve damage, the movement of the small bowel may be disor-dered, leading to stagnation; this allows bacteria to propagate.

Does small bowel bacterial overgrowth cause IBS?

The symptoms of small bowel bacterial overgrowth can be identi-cal to those of IBS, particularly diarrhoea-predominant IBS (IBS-D). Bloating and diarrhoea are prominent in both syndromes. One American study of 111 patients with IBS found evidence of small bowel bacterial overgrowth in 93 (84%) of the patients. Half the patients were treated with an antibiotic and half with an inactive medication (a placebo). About a third (35%) of the patients receiving the antibiotic improved compared with 11% of those who received the placebo. Although this study has not been repeated to confirm it, it does suggest that at least a proportion of patients with IBS have small bowel bacterial overgrowth and will respond to treatment with antibiotics.

But there is much scepticism over this. I frequently treat patients with otherwise unexplained diarrhoea and bloating with antibiotics. In elderly patients, those with diabetes and those who have had surgery on their bowel or stomach, this is often the first therapeutic manoeuvre. A proportion of patients do show a benefit, making the treatment worthwhile, but most do not. You can discuss the possibility of antibiotic treatment with your doctor.

How do I know whether I've got small bowel overgrowth?

There are breath tests that look for the breakdown products of bacterial metabolism excreted in the breath. A sample of the contents of the upper small bowel can also be taken during an endoscopy (in which a tube with a camera is inserted into the gut via the oesophagus; Chapter 13 explains more about this) and tested for bacterial infection. But contamination of the sample by the bacteria in the mouth usually makes the test useless. In fact, all the tests for small bowel bacterial overgrowth can be inaccurate, and the simplest approach is often just to try some treatment.

How can small bowel bacterial overgrowth be treated?

Many antibiotics will work, including metronidazole, ciprofloxacin, tetracycline and Augmentin. There may be a dramatic improvement over a week, although occasionally a month's treatment is necessary. The infection frequently recurs, and further courses of antibiotics are used. Unfortunately, some people need almost continuous treatment with antibiotics. This may involve 2 weeks of ciprofloxacin followed by 2 weeks of metronidazole followed by 2 weeks of tetracycline and so on. Rotating the treatment is a way of keeping the bacteria sensitive to the antibiotics.

I asked my family doctor to prescribe antibiotics for me in case my IBS was due to small bowel bacterial overgrowth. He was willing to do so, but reluctantly and with much scepticism. Why is that?

The infection in small bowel bacterial overgrowth is a mixed infection. Therefore, most antibiotics will reduce the number of infecting bacteria and should improve the symptoms. Antibiotics are very frequently prescribed for many different infections, but we don't generally get people telling us how much better their IBS is since the antibiotic they had for their chest, throat or urine infection. In fact, the opposite is more common: people more often tell us that the antibiotics have exacerbated their IBS. Your doctor would be wary of this happening to you.

GIARDIASIS

Are there other infections that can masquerade as IBS?

Surprisingly, many people have never heard of the organism *Giardia lamblia* even though it is one of the most common parasitic infections in the world. Infection rates may be as high as 2–5% in the industrialised world. A staggering 20–30% of individuals in some regions of the developing world are infected.

Giardia lamblia is a one-celled organism that lives in the small bowel of both animals and humans. It forms cysts that are excreted in the stool, survive in fresh water and are relatively insensitive to chlorination. People become infected from water, food or drinks contaminated by the faeces of other infected people or animals. Many cases are associated with recent foreign travel.

The incubation period is 1–2 weeks, and the most common symptoms are diarrhoea with watery, foul-smelling stools, often with abdominal distension, flatulence, nausea, anorexia and vomiting. Most people will have a minor, self-limiting illness. Others may have a more severe illness and undergo tests, from which *Giardia* is recognised and treated. But in a significant number of people, the symptoms may arise gradually over a few weeks and may be troublesome rather than severe.

These individuals may not go to their doctor. If and when they do ask the doctor for help, the gradual onset of their symptoms and the length of time that they have been troubled tend to argue against an infection and towards a diagnosis of IBS. People complain of loose, watery stools, bloating and excessive offensive flatulence going on for months or even years. They may be absolutely well in themselves, with nothing to suggest an infection or a serious illness. It is therefore easy for patients and their doctors to attribute the symptoms of giardiasis to an irritable bowel.

So does giardiasis cause IBS?

Giardiasis does not cause IBS, but it may be mistaken for it. Many doctors don't appreciate how common it is even in developed societies. This confusion can mean that you may be treated for IBS until the diagnosis of giardiasis becomes apparent.

How is giardiasis diagnosed?

The cysts of *Giardia* may be identified when stool is examined under a microscope. The problem is that the cysts may be excreted intermittently, so that even though an individual is infected, there may be no cysts in the stool. Moreover, the cysts can be difficult to see. Giardiasis can also be diagnosed by biopsies (samples of cells) taken from the duodenum (the part of the intestine that follows on from the stomach; see Figure 1.1) at endoscopy. Here, the *Giardia* organisms are seen lying along the wall of the intestine.

More sophisticated stool tests will become available in the future. In the meantime, it is often better to treat people whenever there is a suspicion of *Giardia*.

If I have giardiasis, how will it be treated?

Giardiasis is usually treated with a 1-week course of the antibiotic metronidazole. The common side effects of this medication are a bitter taste, nausea and vomiting. Alcohol can make these side effects much worse.

A major problem in treating patients with *Giardia* infection is the recurrence of symptoms after standard courses of therapy. This may be due to several causes. First, the organism may be resistant to the treatment, so a longer course of metronidazole may be necessary. Second, the original infection may have been eliminated but the person may have become reinfected. Finally, the infection may have been eliminated, but the individual may be left with lactose intolerance (see an earlier question).

COELIAC DISEASE

This is also known as coeliac sprue or gluten-sensitive enteropathy.

My friend's just been diagnosed with coeliac disease. What is this?

The immune system has a large presence within the gut to protect us from any infection that we might ingest with our food. In coeliac disease, it makes a mistake and mounts a response to a protein constituent of wheat called gluten. Related proteins in rye, barley and possibly oats are also involved. The result is a low level of inflammation in the wall of the small bowel that damages its capacity to digest and absorb food.

The surface of the inner wall of the small bowel is designed so as to maximise its area. There are numerous folds, and the surface is covered by finger-like projections about 0.5–1.5 millimetres long that protrude into the intestinal lumen and are called villi. It is the villi that are principally damaged in coeliac disease. Indeed, they may be completely lost such that the inner surface of the small bowel appears flat. The consequence is a marked loss in surface area, which impairs digestion and absorption.

Although coeliac disease was recognised in ancient times, its association with wheat was only discovered by the Dutch paediatrician W. K. Dicke towards the end of the World War II. At that time, food, particularly the cereals used to make bread, was scarce in The Netherlands. Yet the condition of children with coeliac disease improved. Dr Dicke noticed that these children relapsed when bread was supplied at the end of the war by the Swedish Air Force. It was this serendipitous observation that led to the finding that wheat exacerbates coeliac disease.

Most of the damage is in the upper part of the small bowel, while the lower part of the small bowel may be unaffected. To a certain, but variable, extent, the unaffected small bowel makes up for the reduced function of the upper small bowel. This is one of the reasons why the symptoms of coeliac disease are so variable. Some people have a life-threatening illness with terrible diarrhoea and weight loss. Some have no symptoms at all, whereas others have symptoms that are easily interpreted as an irritable bowel, with bloating, flatulence, loose stools and abdominal pains.

Who gets coeliac disease?

Twenty years ago, we thought of coeliac disease as a rare childhood disorder. Today, we realise that it can become apparent at any age. There is a genetic susceptibility to coeliac disease that may affect as many as 1% of northern European Caucasian populations, but it is rare in people of African/Caribbean or Chinese origin. If you have coeliac disease, there is a 10% chance that your close relatives (parents, siblings and children) will also get the disease.

How is coeliac disease diagnosed?

With modern endoscopes, it is easy to take biopsies (samples) from the upper small bowel. When these are examined under a microscope, they have a loss or flattening of the villi, the finger-like projections on the bowel wall, together with an increase in the number of inflammatory cells. The diagnosis is confirmed by an improvement in symptoms, biopsy appearances or both with a gluten-free diet.

Over the past 20 years, simple and inexpensive blood tests for coeliac disease have been developed and refined. They test for evidence of an immune reaction to gluten by looking for specific antibodies in the blood. The tests are very sensitive, and coeliac disease is unlikely if they are negative. Occasionally, the blood test is positive but the patient does not have coeliac disease. So whenever the blood test is positive, a biopsy of the small bowel is necessary to confirm the diagnosis before treatment is started.

How do you treat coeliac disease?

Coeliac disease is treated with a gluten-free diet. Products containing wheat, rye, barley, and traditionally oats are avoided. The distant cousins of wheat, such as maize, rice and sorghum are safe, as is buckwheat, which is a legume rather than a cereal. Vegetables and meats are completely safe too.

On the face of it, eating a gluten-free diet seems relatively simple, but in practice it can be terribly difficult because wheat products are included in an enormous range of processed foods and may not be mentioned in the labelling. You need to be aware that hidden gluten can be found in some unlikely foods such as cold meat cuts, soups, soy sauce, many low or non-fat products and even licorice and jelly beans. A number of organisations provide regularly updated information about the contents of manufactured foods. Useful contacts include the Celiac Sprue Association of the USA, the Celiac Disease Foundation and Coeliac UK (see the Appendix for details).

Does coeliac disease cause IBS?

No, coeliac disease doesn't cause IBS, but the symptoms of coeliac disease can be identical to those of IBS, especially diarrhoea-predominant IBS (IBS-D). Bloating and diarrhoea are prominent in both syndromes. Because coeliac disease involves the poor digestion and absorption of food, weight loss is an expected symptom and can be severe. By contrast, weight loss is unusual in IBS. Surprisingly, though, many patients with coeliac disease do not lose weight. Indeed, I have diagnosed coeliac disease in severely obese patients! As a result, many doctors will perform a blood test for coeliac disease before diagnosing IBS, just to make sure.

Coeliac disease is, however, frequently misdiagnosed as IBS. In one study, 36% of people with coeliac disease had previously been diagnosed as suffering from IBS.

INFLAMMATORY BOWEL DISEASE

What is inflammatory bowel disease?

The inflammatory bowel diseases are a group of conditions in which inflammation occurs and continues within the gastrointestinal tract. In ulcerative colitis, the inflammation is confined to the large bowel. In Crohn's disease, any part of the gastrointestinal tract can be affected. What causes these conditions is unknown, and although they cannot be cured, they can usually be controlled. The inflammation in these diseases is usually considerably more severe than what is seen in coeliac disease or infections of the bowel. In ulcerative colitis, people commonly report diarrhoea with blood and mucus in the stool. In Crohn's disease, abdominal pain and weight loss can be profound.

Can inflammatory bowel disease be mistaken for IBS – they sound a bit similar?

The symptoms of inflammatory bowel disease can come on slowly over weeks or months. There may be a little abdominal pain, the stools may become a little loose, and people may feel somewhat tired. It is easy for them to interpret these symptoms as 'an infection that will pass' or as IBS. In contrast to IBS, however, the symptoms of inflammatory bowel disease do get worse. Diarrhoea occurring at night, weight loss and bleeding are also clues that the diagnosis is unlikely to be IBS and should prompt people to seek medical attention.

Can inflammatory bowel disease cause IBS?

Unfortunately, inflammatory bowel disease is frequently complicated by IBS. It is a real problem, affecting up to half of people with ulcerative colitis or Crohn's disease. In inflammatory bowel disease, there is excessive inflammation in the intestine, causing diarrhoea, bleeding and pain. This inflammation can usually be successfully treated by medication, but unfortunately even when the inflammation is completely suppressed, people may continue to have IBS-type symptoms. It can be difficult to know if the loose stools, bloating and pain represent a recurrence of the inflammation or an irritable bowel following it.

In ulcerative colitis, the inflammation begins at the rectum, so it is fairly straightforward to perform a limited examination of the rectum to gauge the degree of inflammation. In Crohn's disease, however, the inflammation can be anywhere in the gut, and a full examination of the entire gut is a major undertaking. Moreover, blood tests in Crohn's disease can be normal even during a severe exacerbation. So whether the symptoms represent an exacerbation of inflammatory bowel disease or IBS is often a matter of judgement. Treatment, as in many conditions may come down to experimentation to find what works best for you.

I've suffered from ulcerative colitis affecting just my rectum for many years, and I've always had a problem with diarrhoea, especially in the morning. My doctors tell me that there is now no active inflammation, but I've still got bad diarrhoea. What can I do? I've tried loperamide in the past and it didn't work.

Loperamide does not work well when there is inflammation, but it may work extremely well when the colitis is in remission and there is no or little inflammation. If your diarrhoea is mainly in the morning, you can try one or two capsules of loperamide before going to bed.

. . . No, the loperamide didn't work for me. And my doctor's said that after many years of ulcerative colitis in the rectum, I now have a 'micro rectum'. What does she mean?

She means that your rectum does not distend (expand) enough to hold the stool. As the normal rectum fills with stool, it expands so that the pressure within it remains more or less constant. Only when it is full does the pressure rise, sending us the message that we need to go to the toilet. In some people, after many years of inflammation in the rectum, the wall becomes damaged and will not stretch to accommodate the stool. So even a small amount of stool entering the rectum can elicit a 'call to stool'.

DIETARY FIBRE AND DIARRHOEA

You hear so much about dietary fibre these days. What exactly is it?

Dietary fibre is indigestible plant carbohydrate (mainly substances known as cellulose, pectins and lignins from the plant cell wall). It passes through the small bowel undigested to the large bowel where bacteria partially metabolise it into gas, liquid and short-chain fatty acids. The short-chain fatty acids are absorbed by the large bowel; these are an important nutrient for us. Most of what is left passes through the gut in the stool, along with water and gas trapped within it and bacteria growing on it. Fibre therefore produces a softer, wetter, bulkier stool that is easier to pass.

I have diarrhoea-predominant IBS. Should I eat more dietary fibre?

If your diarrhoea is actually caused by constipation and overflow (Chapter 7 explains what this is), more fibre may help. It may also help if you have alternating constipation and diarrhoea (see Chapter 9). However, since fibre holds water within your bowel, it is inevitable that, regardless of the underlying cause, more fibre will mean more diarrhoea.

MEDICATION THAT SLOWS THE BOWEL

Currently, the most potent drugs for slowing the bowel and relaxing its muscle are opiate based. 'Opiate' refers to drugs originally produced from the immature seed capsules of the opium poppy plant. Our nervous system produces its own opiate-like chemicals called endorphins. Their principal role is to reduce pain, and many of the cells involved in pain processing have receptors for the endorphin molecules on their surface. These receptors also interact with opiate drugs, so they've been called opiate receptors.

In the bowel, however, activation of the opiate receptors leads to relaxation of the bowel muscle and a profound slowing in function. This is why opiate-based analgesics (painkillers) such as codeine and morphine can cause severe constipation, and why opiate-based drugs can relieve diarrhoea. You can find information on these opiate agents in Table 8.3.

Table 8.3 Opiate medications used to treat diarrhoea

Drug	Trade names	Comment
Loperamide	Arrett Capsules, Boots Diareze, Diasorb, Diocalm Ultra, Imodium (including Imodium liquid), Imodium Plus and Normaloe	This is an opiate-based drug that acts selectively on the gut. As a result, it has little or no analgesic effect. There is also little or no risk of dependence. Drowsiness may be a side effect in large doses, but most people are virtually unaffected. A single dose of loperamide can remain effective for 24 hours
Diphenoxylate and atropine	Lomotil	Diphenoxylate is similar to loperamide. The small dose of atropine in the mixture also slows the bowel by blocking the activity of another set of nerves (cholinergic nerves) that would otherwise increase bowel activity. In larger doses, atropine will cause unpleasant side effects such as a dry mouth and blurred vision. This means that Lomotil cannot be taken in large doses
Codeine and dihydrocodeine	These are available over the counter in small doses, usually combined with paracetamol	These are opiate-based medications used mainly as analgesics. They slow the bowel effectively, but are likely to cause drowsiness. Tolerance is a problem, which means they may become less effective over time. It is possible to become addicted to codeine

Loperamide and IBS

Loperamide is one of the few medications used in IBS for which there is clear evidence that it is effective. It is usually very good when used to reduce or prevent diarrhoea. Usually, only small doses – one or two capsules a day – are necessary, sometimes even fewer. If your diarrhoea does not respond to loperamide, it may not be due to IBS. Loperamide is safe to use in the long term, and the only significant side effect is constipation.

Loperamide is not an analgesic, which means that it is ineffective for pain. But sometimes the pain in IBS is due to excessive muscular activity and spasm in the wall of the bowel. In such circumstances, loperamide may help.

Can loperamide make IBS worse?

People with IBS are often very sensitive to the effects of loperamide. A small dose can result in constipation with increased bloating and painful spasm. A loperamide syrup is available for children, but adults can use it to take very small doses.

What about Dioralyte? Could this help stop my diarrhoea?

Dioralyte is one of the oral rehydration salts available at pharmacies. Others include Rehidrat and Electrolade. They come as sachets of powder or effervescent tablets that are reconstituted with water. They contain sodium chloride (salt), potassium and bicarbonate, along with glucose to stimulate the absorption of these. Their purpose is to replace the water and minerals lost in severe infective diarrhoea.

The rationale behind this treatment is that some people with diarrhoea will only drink water. But drinking just water does not replace the salt and potassium lost in the diarrhoea, and moreover water taken on its own may not be well absorbed. Glucose not only acts as an energy source but actually stimulates the absorption of salt and water in the small bowel. A solution of glucose with salt, potassium and bicarbonate, with some flavouring to make it reasonably palatable, has proved very successful as a readily available, safe and cheap method of rehydrating people with severe infective diarrhoea, especially in the developing world.

Unfortunately, oral rehydrating solutions will not stop or reduce your diarrhoea. Their function is to replace the fluids and minerals that are lost. Personally, I prefer chicken soup.

My mother used to give me a liquid called Kaolin and Morphine whenever I had diarrhoea. What does it do, and is it still available?

Kaolin is a clay material traditionally used to soothe the stomach and the bowels. It is believed to absorb excess water, toxins and possibly bacteria, although this has never been formally tested. It is still available without prescription as Kaolin Light, or combined with a small dose of morphine. The morphine will reduce pain from spasm and slow the bowel down. Although it is present only in small amounts, there is a risk of drowsiness. As a treatment for diarrhoea, it is not as effective as loperamide.

An American friend has recommended bismuth subsalicylate for diarrhoea. What is it, and does it work?

Bismuth is a silvery metallic element whose compounds are used for various stomach and bowel problems and are still popular. It is believed that bismuth compounds may form protective coatings for inflamed surfaces such as ulcers. Bismuth itself may have antibacterial properties and has been used to protect against travellers' diarrhoea. The subsalicylate portion of bismuth subsalicylate may improve diarrhoea by promoting absorption. It is available in the UK as Pepto-Bismol. For diarrhoea, it is not as effective as loperamide, and a large dose needs to be taken (30–60 ml or 2–4 tablets every 30 minutes up to eight doses). It causes temporary and harmless staining of your tongue, but don't get it on your carpet!

PROBLEMS AND SOLUTIONS

Food passes straight through me. Whenever I eat, I feel a violent need to rush to the toilet to pass a loose stool. It's very embarrassing as well as inconvenient. Despite this diarrhoea, I can't lose weight. What's happening?

This may not be true diarrhoea. You are actually describing a strong gastrocolic reflex. A reflex is an unconscious automatic response in which stimulation of one part of the body results in activity in another. For example, tapping the tendon under your knee leads to a reflex contraction of your thigh muscle, and your foot goes up. In the gut, filling and distension (expansion) of the stomach leads to nervous impulses that stimulate activity in the bowel. This is a normal reflex. It is stronger in some people than others, and it is often more prominent if you have IBS or inflammatory bowel disease.

The simplest way of controlling this is to eat smaller meals, or to eat more slowly in order to reduce the distension of the stomach. Eating less fat may help too. Fatty foods tend to slow the emptying of the stomach, so a fatty meal will tend to distend the stomach more. You may also wish to avoid taking caffeine with your meal as it will increase the stimulation of your bowel.

Sometimes taking an antispasmodic medication such as peppermint oil or alverine citrate (Spasmonal) before your meals may help. These are usually available at the chemist without a prescription. A more potent alternative available on prescription is dicycloverine (dicyclomine, Merbentyl), which reduces spasm and slows the bowel down. Loperamide (Imodium) is good at slowing the bowel, and some people with a prominent gastrocolic reflex take a capsule before going out for a big meal.

I get sudden episodes of diarrhoea, especially when I'm stressed or rushing for the airport. What can I do?

If you can predict the circumstances in which your bowels may be overactive, you can take a loperamide (Imodium) capsule at an appropriate time, such as before going out.

I get diarrhoea at night as well as during the day. I have to get up several times during the night, and my sleep is badly disturbed. What can I do?

Diarrhoea at night is very unusual in IBS. It is likely that there is a cause other than IBS for your problem and you should see your doctor.

My main problem is first thing in the morning. The moment I wake up, I have to rush to the bathroom. The first bits I pass may be solid, but after that I have to rush several times to pass watery stools. What can I do?

This is a very common manifestation of IBS. You could try a loperamide (Imodium) capsule before going to bed, or first thing in the morning.

I've tried loperamide, but even just one capsule will stop me going for several days! That can't be good for me, and it's certainly uncomfortable. What can I do?

People with IBS are often very sensitive to loperamide. It's a particular problem for those who have alternating constipation and diarrhoea (see Chapter 9). But Imodium syrup might help. This contains 1 mg of loperamide in each 5 ml dose, or the equivalent of half a capsule per spoonful. It's then possible to take very small doses. Alternatively, you could try a small dose of Lomotil.

I've tried to slow my bowel down with loperamide, but it only works if I take eight or more capsules a day. I've also tried codeine, Lomotil and kaolin, but again they only work partially even in large doses. What should I do?

Your diarrhoea may not be due to IBS. People with IBS are usually very sensitive to medication that slows the bowel, such as loperamide. If loperamide doesn't work, you should see your doctor to consider other diagnoses.

I've suffered from IBS for many years. Some days I get diarrhoea, then at other times I'm constipated, and occasionally I'm OK. Over the last 3 months, things have changed so that I get diarrhoea all the time. It isn't so bad that I can't control it with loperamide, but I'm 65 years old and concerned about the change. What ought I to do?

You should see your doctor. There may be an obvious explanation such as a change in your diet or a new medication. However, if there is any doubt, an examination of your bowel to exclude cancer is important.

I'm only 32 years old. How concerned should I be about a change in my bowel habit? Like many people with IBS, some days I get diarrhoea, but at other times I'm constipated. Over the past few months, things have changed so that I now get diarrhoea all the time unless I take one or two capsules of loperamide each day.

If you can control your bowels with one or two capsules of loperamide a day, it's unlikely that your symptoms are anything other than IBS. There may or may not be an obvious explanation such as a change in your diet or a new medication. But at your age, bowel cancer is very unlikely. If there is no weight loss, anaemia or bleeding, and no family history of bowel cancer, your bowel does not need to be examined.

. . . Yes, I understand what you are saying, but I can't get the thought of cancer out of my head. I like my doctor, but I'm afraid he will laugh at me if I say I'm frightened about this. What should I do?

Doctors don't usually laugh at patients; we prefer to laugh at other doctors! Physicians laugh at general surgeons, general surgeons laugh at orthopaedic surgeons, orthopaedic surgeons laugh at ..., and so on. You would probably be surprised at how much understanding you get if you directly express your fear of cancer or any other disease. Most doctors, surrounded by illness as they are, have at one time or another thought they had a serious ailment. If your doctor laughs, he is more likely to be laughing with you than at you as he'll have been there himself. So do go and book an appointment so that you can set your mind at rest.

My diarrhoea didn't respond to any treatment. I had many tests, including a colonoscopy, all of which were normal. Finally, my doctor suggested cholestyramine (Questran). It worked! I've been told that my diarrhoea was due to primary bile acid malabsorption. What is that?

Bile acids are produced in the liver from cholesterol and secreted into the small bowel in the bile. Their function is to help dissolve, digest and absorb fat. In the last part of the small bowel, the terminal ileum, these bile acids are reabsorbed. They travel in the circulation back to the liver to be secreted again in the bile. But some people don't reabsorb the bile acids well enough in the terminal ileum so that they pass into the large bowel. Here, they reduce the ability of the large bowel to absorb water and may actually stimulate it to secrete water. The consequence is a watery diarrhoea that may not respond well to antidiarrhoeal drugs like loperamide.

This failure of the terminal ileum to absorb the bile acids may be due to a disease such as Crohn's disease. It also occasionally happens after a cholecystectomy (excision of the gall bladder), or it may be primary. By primary, we mean that we don't know why it has occurred, and that it is not secondary to (a result of) anything else. Because all the usual tests are normal, the diarrhoea may mistakenly be attributed to IBS.

Cholestyramine binds bile acids to make an inert complex. This complex passes through into the large bowel, where it has no effect at all. Cholestyramine was originally developed as a treatment for high cholesterol levels. As the bile acids are lost from the body when someone takes it, the liver is forced to produce a new supply. It uses cholesterol for this so the blood cholesterol level falls.

The problem with using cholestyramine is knowing how much to use. Too little and it is ineffective. Use too much and too many bile acids are lost. It then becomes difficult to digest fat. If fat is not absorbed, it passes out in the stool, causing a foul-smelling, yellow diarrhoea. It is really a matter of experimenting. I usually advise people to start with half a sachet of cholestyramine at night and increase this by half a sachet every 3 days or so depending on the response. If there is no improvement with one sachet four times a day, then it isn't going to work and the diagnosis isn't bile acid malabsorption.

As a tip, cholestyramine is more palatable if mixed with orange juice.

Recently, I decided to improve my diet by eating more fruit. I eat oranges, pears, grapes and apples. But instead of feeling well, my bowels have become loose, I feel bloated, and I pass a lot of wind. Why has this happened?

There are several possibilities. These fruits contain significant amounts of fructose. If you have an impaired absorption of fructose (an earlier question in this chapter discusses this), that would explain your symptoms. Or your loose stools might simply be a consequence of your increased fibre intake. It could also be just a coincidence, so the first thing to do is see if your bowel habit returns to normal when you revert to your old diet.

After many, many years of suffering from what I took to be IBS,
they finally diagnosed coeliac disease. I've been on a gluten-free
diet for 3 months now, and I can't believe how much better I feel.
I'm still angry though that it took so long to diagnose my
coeliac disease.

It used to be very difficult to diagnose coeliac disease. Twenty years ago, there were no specific blood tests for it. Hence, there was no simple screening test as there is today.

Moreover, if coeliac disease was suspected, proving the diagnosis meant getting the person concerned to swallow a large capsule attached to a long tube and waiting for the capsule to reach the small bowel. The capsule could then be activated to take one small biopsy (sample) and would have to be retrieved by pulling on the tube to which it was attached. It could take a whole day to get a specimen! Nowadays, getting a biopsy from the small bowel involves a gastroscopy (a telescopic examination of the stomach, explained more in Chapter 13), which is usually straightforward. It's probably because coeliac disease was so difficult to diagnose that we only recognised the more extreme cases.

Today, we realise that people with coeliac disease can have a wide range of symptoms. We usually test for coeliac disease with a blood test when people report loose stools, excess wind, bloating, weight loss or fatigue. Although patients with coeliac disease tend to be thin, it has been diagnosed in people who are actually obese. It is likely that there are many people who put up with symptoms that they attribute to IBS when in fact they have coeliac disease.

It's good that your doctor recognised the possibility of coeliac disease masquerading as IBS. As more and more doctors do so, there will less delay in diagnosing coeliac disease in the future.

I thought I had coeliac disease, but the tests were negative.
Even so, I put myself on a gluten-free diet, avoiding anything
that contained wheat or barley. Giving up bread was a major
sacrifice, but I feel enormously better. I no longer have
diarrhoea, I don't bloat nearly as much, and I get a lot less
noise from my stomach. Could the tests have been mistaken?

Unfortunately, no test is perfect. However, it is unusual for people with a negative blood test to turn out later to have coeliac disease. It is even more unusual for biopsies (samples) from the small bowel to miss a diagnosis of coeliac disease. It can happen, though, and we do occasionally repeat the tests.

But there are other possible explanations for why you are feeling so much better on a gluten-free diet even if you do not actually have coeliac disease. A gluten-free diet often means eating less fibre. Some patients with IBS, particularly those who have mainly diarrhoea, feel much better with less fibre in their diet. If this is so in your case, you may be able to eat bread again if you reduce your intake of fibre from other sources.

Alternatively, some people with IBS are simply intolerant of wheat and wheat products. We don't know why an intolerance like this develops, but in contrast to coeliac disease it is not due to an activation of the immune system. Moreover, eating wheat may cause symptoms but it does not cause any damage or long-term harm. So people who are intolerant of wheat but do not have coeliac disease don't need to be as strict with their diet as people with coeliac disease. In fact, they should experiment from time to time with wheat products to see if the intolerance is persisting and how much wheat they can actually tolerate.

I suffered from diarrhoea and had a colonoscopy. They told me it was all normal, but when I came back for a follow-up appointment, I was told that actually the biopsies showed microscopic colitis. What is that?

Microscopic colitis is a colitis that is only diagnosed when biopsy specimens from the bowel are examined under the microscope and show excess inflammation. This colitis is mild, and without a microscope the wall of the bowel looks normal. It may represent a mild form of ulcerative colitis with no ulcers and hence no bleeding, or it may represent another form of colitis such as what are called lymphocytic colitis and collagenous colitis. These disorders usually show up in middle age with persisting watery diarrhoea. They do not progress to anything more serious and are usually treated with a type of anti-inflammatory medication called mesalazine.

. . . Yes, I was treated with mesalazine. But it didn't work. They had another look at my bowel, and this time they told me that my bowel looked normal. They took a lot more biopsies, and they were also normal. So now they're saying that I don't have microscopic colitis, it must be IBS after all! What's going on?

The diagnosis of microscopic colitis depends on a somewhat subjective assessment of the degree of inflammation in the biopsy specimens. A second look, with more biopsies, can clarify the diagnosis.

It is also possible that the original microscopic inflammation was due to a previous infection. This infection has now cleared but left you with an irritable bowel. This is called postinfective irritable bowel syndrome (IBS-PI). In surveys, about 10% of people with an irritable bowel recall an infection that seemed to set off their IBS. In studies of previously well people diagnosed with bacterial gastroenteritis, 7–31% developed an irritable bowel in the 3–6 months after the infection. Gastroenteritis, either viral or bacterial, is an important cause of IBS. The diarrhoea is usually easily controlled with loperamide.

How long does postinfective irritable bowel last?

There isn't much information with which to answer this question, but one study suggests that 6 years after a diagnosis of postinfective IBS, fewer than half of the people affected had recovered.

FAECAL INCONTINENCE

I sometimes need to really rush to the toilet. I get a spasm in the lower part of my abdomen on the left, and I know that if I don't reach a toilet quickly, I will mess myself. It can happen at any time, but it usually happens on the way to work. Most of the time I'm OK, but the fear of soiling myself in public has come to haunt me. I've tried taking Imodium, but it just makes me constipated, and then it's all worse. What can I do?

Having to rush to the toilet is called 'urgency of stool'. This is common in IBS, but it is usually intermittent, occurring mainly in the morning rather than at night. If your urgency does not settle with the simple measures such as taking a small dose of loperamide, it's possible that there is a more serious problem than IBS irritating the rectum. You should see a doctor with a view to having a telescopic examination of your rectum (called flexible sigmoidoscopy – see Chapter 13 for more information on this) to see whether there is inflammation in the wall of your rectum (colitis) or even a polyp (a small mushroom-like growth, usually not yet malignant) or a tumour.

As you have discovered, it's important to avoid constipation. If your rectum is full, it's much more likely to spasm and force you to rush to the toilet. Ideally, you should have an empty rectum before leaving home in the morning. This means giving yourself enough time. It may mean having breakfast and waiting long enough before leaving home for your bowel to empty. Filling your stomach with food or drink is a natural way to stimulate your bowels to work. It is called the gastrocolic reflex and involves a subconscious message from the stomach to the brain informing the brain that the stomach is full, followed by a message from the brain to the bowel increasing its muscular activity. In some people it is a strong reflex, particularly in the morning, in others it hardly exists.

> *... I've tried to give myself enough time before and after breakfast. I may go several times, but I still get caught short half way to work! What can I do?*

You can try taking a glycerine or bisacodyl suppository when you get up. They work quite quickly and will help to clear the rectum. If one or other isn't enough, you can try both together. The glycerine will draw water into your rectum and elicit a call to stool, while the bisacodyl will stimulate the rectal muscles to clear the rectum.

If suppositories are not effective enough, you can use an enema. Sodium citrate enemas (Micralax and Relaxit Micro-enema) are available without prescription. They come in single-dose disposable packs with a nozzle. Each dose is only 5 ml (about one teaspoonful) of liquid. They are effective and work quickly.

This may sound rather drastic but it is better than being caught short. Moreover, with time, this approach may habituate your bowel to clearing itself in the morning such that you no longer require the suppositories.

> *I can empty my rectum with a suppository, but I still get a terrible urge to go to the toilet on the way to work. I hold on, and by the time I get to work, there is little or nothing to pass. Even so, it can make my journey a nightmare. I'm always afraid of soiling myself.*

It may be that your bowel is simply very active in the morning or that is has somehow got into the habit of reacting this way to the stress and tension of the start of the day. In either case, you can try to reduce spasm with antispasmodic medication such as dicyclover-ine (dicyclomine) or mebeverine (these require a prescription in most countries), or plant extracts such as alverine citrate or peppermint oil, which are usually available over the counter. The most effective solution might be to clear your rectum with a suppository and then take loperamide before going out. But this does run the risk of making you constipated and perpetuating the problem.

Would changing the fibre content of my diet help?

Some people find that bulking up their stool with extra fibre does give them more control and less spasm. Others find that more fibre makes their diarrhoea worse, sometimes much worse. It's a matter of experimenting. Eating less fibre may well give you harder stools, which are easier to hold in, but on the other hand if you become constipated, the whole problem could be much worse. It is also worth trying to avoid stimulants to the bowel such as caffeine. Caffeine is present in coffee and to a lesser extent in tea, cola drinks and chocolate.

I frequently feel the need to go to the toilet urgently, but I only pass small soft or sometimes hard pellets. And despite the urgency, I actually have to strain fairly hard to get them out. It never feels like I have cleared my rectum. What can I do?

You may have a sensitive rectum in which even the minimal distension caused by a small pellet of stool makes you feel you want to go to the toilet urgently. We all find it difficult to pass small pellets, and it's never satisfying. You may well improve with more fibre in your diet. Extra fibre will change pellet-like stools to more sausage-shaped stools, which are easier to pass and more satisfying.

*I don't get diarrhoea as such, but I do leak small amounts of
stool and mucus. It's terribly irritating as well as embarrassing.
What can I do?*

F irming up your stool with small doses of loperamide will probably
help. Loperamide also tightens the anal sphincter – the muscle
that stops stool leaking out.

A weak anal sphincter may be your problem. It may be weakened
with age, but giving birth is the most common cause of damage. One
study has demonstrated that over a third of women have damage to
their anal sphincter after their first vaginal delivery. If the delivery is
difficult and forceps are used, up to 80% may have damage to their
anal sphincter. The consequence is faecal leakage in later life. It usually isn't severe, but even a little can be very irritating and disruptive.

Is there anything I can do to strengthen my anal sphincter?

You can try to strengthen your anal sphincter by exercising it. This
means repeatedly tightening and relaxing your anus. The sphincter
is a muscle, and just like any other muscle, it should strengthen with
exercise. In fact, if you want to tighten your anal sphincter, it's necessary to work all the muscles in your pelvic floor. So this exercise is
recommended for women with stress incontinence (leakage of urine
occurring with normal physical activity such as laughing, coughing,
lifting or other exercise) and for men with incontinence following
prostate surgery, as well as for people with faecal leakage. It is also
said to improve sexual function in women by strengthening the vaginal muscles. In the USA, pelvic floor exercises are called Kegel
exercises after their originator, Dr Arnold Kegel.

What do pelvic floor (Kegel) exercises feel like?

F irst, sit on the toilet and start to urinate. Try to stop the flow of
urine in midstream by contracting your pelvic floor muscles. Try
not to contract your abdominal, thigh or buttock muscles – they

should remain relaxed. Repeat this action several times until you become familiar with the feel of contracting the correct group of muscles.

Some people find this exercise very easy to do, whereas others have a problem identifying the group of muscles that form the pelvic floor and keep contracting their abdominal wall or thigh muscles. Another approach is to place a finger in the rectum or vagina and to tighten your muscles around it, squeezing against the resistance of the finger, holding and then releasing.

This is called an isometric exercise. In this, the length of the muscle is unchanged but the exercise increases the tone of the muscle, so it's tighter at rest. The strength of the muscle contraction is also increased, allowing a better control of urinary or faecal urgency.

A woman may also strengthen these muscles by using a vaginal cone, which is a weighted device that is inserted into her vagina. She can then try to contract the pelvic floor muscles in an effort to hold the device the place.

I have heard of biofeedback as a treatment for incontinence. What exactly does it involve?

For those people who are unsure whether they are performing the procedure correctly, biofeedback and electrical stimulation may be used to help to identify the correct muscle group to work on. Biofeedback is a method of positive reinforcement. Electrodes are placed on the abdomen and along the anal area. Some therapists place a sensor in the vagina if the person is a woman, or the anus if a man, to monitor the contraction of the pelvic floor muscles. A monitor displays a graph showing which muscles are contracting and which are at rest. The therapist can then help to identify the correct muscles for performing pelvic floor exercises. Simple biofeedback equipment can be purchased for use at home.

Electrical stimulation involves using low-voltage electric current to stimulate the correct group of muscles. The current may be delivered using an anal or vaginal probe. The electrical stimulation therapy may be performed in the clinic or at home. The electrical stimulation helps the patient feel which muscles she should be working. The monitors will show her if she is working the right muscle groups, and by trial and error help her learn to better control them.

Simple biofeedback equipment can be purchased for use at home. The electrical current is just strong enough to cause muscles to contract but below the level that would cause pain. There is thus minimal if any discomfort. Once the woman has learnt to perform the exercises correctly, the biofeedback equipment is no longer necessary.

How much should I exercise my pelvic floor?

There are different recommendations, but essentially the more you do, the more likely you are to improve. You can do these exercises any time and anywhere – no one needs to know, and no one will notice.

You should do two kinds of pelvic floor exercises: short squeezes and long squeezes. To do the short squeezes, tighten your pelvic floor muscles quickly, squeeze hard for 2 seconds and then relax the muscle. To do the long squeezes, tighten the muscle for 5–10 seconds before you relax. Do both of these exercises 40–50 times each day.

How long will it take for these exercises to make a difference?

Some people will improve within a couple of weeks, whereas with others it may take 6 weeks or more. You should plan on continuing the exercises for at least 6–12 weeks. Sadly, not everyone will improve even with biofeedback.

ITCHY ANUS (PRURITUS ANI)

Why do I get a terrible itching in my anus?

There are many possible causes of this, and it's very common in people with loose stools or incontinence of the stools. The skin of the anus is easily irritated by frequent wiping. Tiny amounts of faeces repeatedly contaminate the sore skin around the anus, leading to more irritation. This itching is almost impossible to resist, and we can even scratch unconsciously in our sleep. The scratching damages the skin even more, leading to soreness. Healing is then associated with itching, and an itch–scratch cycle develops. The skin never gets chance to heal properly, so the problem continues.

How should I look after my anus?

First of all, **keep it clean and dry**. Wash the skin with water after each stool whenever possible. You may wish to carry a small bottle of water with you when you are out or at work. At least, moisten the toilet paper with water and be gentle. Pat the skin dry, and do not rub it, however tempting this may be. Some people with hairy bottoms use a hair-drier. Wear loose clothing and avoid nylon to reduce sweating.

Next, **avoid irritants**. Soaps and scents can irritate the skin. Spicy foods, tomatoes and fruit can also cause anal irritation in some people. Along with other high-fibre foods, they can cause loose stools and flatulence that will make anal hygiene more difficult.

Finally, you can try **creams and ointments**. Many creams and ointments are available to soothe the anus. Most are marketed for treating haemorrhoids (piles), but they will also help with itching and soreness. Those containing a local anaesthetic (such as lignocaine) are especially effective. Unfortunately, it is possible to become sensitised to one or more of the ingredients in these preparations, especially to the local anaesthetic. Once you are sensitised, the cream only gives temporary relief and may exacerbate the problem by causing dermatitis (eczema) in the anal area. It is worth using these preparations for a few days to a week when the problem starts or if it is severe, to help you interrupt the itch–scratch cycle.

What's the difference between a cream and an ointment?

Creams are a mixture of oil and water, whereas ointments contain no water and are just grease based. This difference is important. Because of their water content, creams must contain preservatives, to which our skin can become sensitive. Creams are more absorbable and wash off easily, whereas ointments leave a greasy layer on the skin. Ointments will therefore offer more protection to the anal skin from irritants in the stool, moisture and friction. The choice of ointment or cream is one of personal comfort, but if you have a difficult or persisting problem, an ointment is probably better both to protect the skin and to avoid preservatives.

Which cream or ointment should I use?

It's perfectly all right to use an ointment or a cream with local anaesthetic in to relieve the torture of anal soreness or itching. Use whichever preparation you find most comfortable; most are available without prescription. But bear in mind that your skin can become sensitised to these preparations within weeks or days, so try and use them for as short a time as possible and concentrate on anal hygiene. If you need to use something, get as bland a preparation as possible. Petroleum jelly (Vaseline) or the creams and ointments produced to prevent nappy rash in babies may also work in adults.

What about steroid-containing ointments?

These can be useful to break the itch–scratch cycle or help anal dermatitis (eczema). They should be for short-term use only, otherwise they will thin and damage the skin.

I have a terrible problem with anal itching at night. What can I do?

You can try a sedating antihistamine tablet before bed. Chlorphenamine (Piriton) is available without prescription. It will reduce itching and help you sleep (the sedative effect). It can be used in the long term and is not addictive.

You may also scratch in your sleep without realising. To help this, wear loose cotton briefs at night to reduce your unconscious access to your anus, keep your fingernails short to limit any damage done to the skin and consider wearing cotton gloves at night to prevent sharp scratching with the fingernails.

. . . I've tried all of these things but I still have a terrible problem with anal itching. What should I do?

It's worth seeing your doctor. There are other possible causes of anal itching, including skin conditions such as eczema or psoriasis, infections such as threadworms or thrush, and occasionally anal tumours.

What are threadworms?

Threadworms are small intestinal worm parasites. The female worm lays many tiny eggs around the anus, and around the vagina and urethra in girls. This usually happens at night, when the infested person is asleep. When laying the eggs, the female worm also secretes an irritant mucus, which causes the person to scratch the itchy area. The eggs then stick under the fingernails and on the fingertips, and can be transferred to the mouth to cause reinfestation. The worms may be seen in the stool or on the anus and look like threads of cotton about 2–13 millimetres long.

Threadworm infection is most common in young children and can be prevented or treated by strict hygiene. A single dose of the medication mebendazole will kill all the worms; it can be purchased without a prescription.

I'm very embarrassed by this problem. Do you have any other advice?

Good advice sheets are available on the Internet – for example, at www.patient.co.uk or www.prodigy.nhs.uk – or by searching for pruritus ani via a search engine such as Google.

CONCLUSION

In terms of comfort and long-term health, it is probably marginally better to be on the loose side than to be constipated. It certainly does no harm to be loose, or even to have frank diarrhoea, providing you drink enough to keep well hydrated. But it can be inconvenient and may lead to a sore anus. Diarrhoea in IBS usually responds to small doses of loperamide. If it does not, the diagnosis should be reconsidered. Weight loss, night-time diarrhoea and blood in the stools are *not* features of IBS and should prompt investigation for more serious pathology. An urgent need to go to the toilet, especially if there is any faecal leakage or anal irritation, can be particularly troublesome. There are several approaches to try and you should not be embarrassed to ask for advice.

SUMMARY

- About one third of people with IBS have diarrhoea as one of their main problems (IBS-D).

- A number of conditions can masquerade as IBS-D, including lactose intolerance, fructose intolerance, coeliac disease, small bowel bacterial overgrowth, mild inflammatory bowel disease and giardiasis.

- Diarrhoea in IBS is usually easily controlled with small doses of loperamide.

- Diarrhoea occurring at night is unlikely to be due to IBS.

■ Diarrhoea associated with involuntary weight loss is unlikely to be due to IBS.

■ A change in bowel habit to looser, more frequent stools in a person over the age of 50 should be investigated to exclude bowel cancer, which is a possible cause.

■ Pelvic floor exercises are the key to controlling incontinence but need to be continued for at least 6 weeks.

■ Consult your doctor. Your local hospital may have a Nurse Continence Advisor.

■ Anal cleanliness is the key to controlling anal itching.

9 | Alternating diarrhoea and constipation

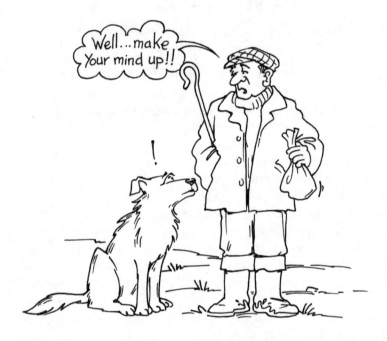

Irritable bowel syndrome (IBS) can be classified into four subgroups: diarrhoea predominant (IBS-D), constipation predominant (IBS-C) and alternating diarrhoea and constipation (IBS-A), occasionally also referred to as IBS-M, for mixed diarrhoea and constipation. In surveys, about a quarter to a third of people fall into each group. The fourth category is referred to 'Unsubtyped IBS' (IBS-U), denoting people with IBS symptoms but with insufficient change in the character of their stools to fit into any of the other categories.

Most treatments for IBS are designed to control either diarrhoea or constipation. People in the IBS-A group have the most variable symptoms. They don't fit easily into treatment groups for research studies, so there is little research into the best way of alleviating their symptoms. If you have IBS-A, you should probably begin by reading Chapters 7 and 8 on constipation and diarrhoea, respectively, as you may like to try some of the strategies outlined for both problems.

Does each subtype of IBS denote a different disease?

The subtype of IBS does not seem to be related to any known aetiology (cause). For example, IBS that follows gastrointestinal infections (postinfective IBS) can present as any of the three subtypes. Visceral hypersensitivity (the concept of enhanced perception, or enhanced responsiveness within the gut – even to normal events; see Chapter 4) can be demonstrated in all IBS subtypes.

Are people fixed into one type of IBS?

The character of IBS symptoms changes with time. Indeed, it is likely that most people will be found to be alternating between diarrhoea and constipation if they are studied for long enough. The IBS-A subgroup may actually be a transition group between IBS-D and IBS-C.

How frequently do people with IBS-A alternate between diarrhoea and constipation?

About a third of people alternate between hard, lumpy and looser, watery bowel motions within a 24-hour period. Another third alternate within a few days. Fewer than 10% alternate over a few weeks, but with the rest there is no pattern at all.

Which is worse for long-term health – constipation or diarrhoea?

It is probably better to keep the bowel clear, but the detrimental effects of constipation have been greatly exaggerated in the past.

PROBLEMS AND SOLUTIONS

I have IBS-A. What treatment should I take?

If you have sustained periods of diarrhoea or constipation, you could use treatments appropriate to those subtypes, for example laxatives when you are constipated, and loperamide when you have diarrhoea.

My IBS symptoms alter during the day. I might pass a hard stool in the morning, and then loose stools through the day. What should I do?

There are a number of alternatives that you should consider. It's possible that the underlying problem is constipation. Your hard stool in the morning may be part of an incomplete evacuation, while the subsequent 'diarrhoea' is the bowel's attempt to clear itself. Secreted water is bypassing hard stool. This is called overflow diarrhoea and is surprisingly common. The solution is to take stimulant laxatives such as senna or bisacodyl in large doses for a few days to really clear your bowel. You do this as a therapeutic experiment. If, with the laxatives, you pass a lot of stool and then feel better for a week or two, you have a strategy that you can use whenever necessary, while concentrating on avoiding constipation.

Alternatively, you may need to choose which symptoms are least and most disturbing to you. You may feel more comfortable with an empty bowel, and might feel you can put up with the diarrhoea. In that case take a laxative, or more fibre. Alternatively, if it's the diarrhoea that it is most disturbing, take loperamide at low doses. With the loperamide, you may get very constipated and have to accept that every so often you will have to stop taking it for a few days and even take some laxatives to clear your bowel.

A further alternative for you is to use a glycerine or bisacodyl suppository in the morning to help with the hard stool and evacuate as much as possible. If you can get a clear rectum, you may have a great deal less trouble with urgent bowel motions during the rest of the day. It is also reasonable to clear your rectum with a suppository, and then once your bowels have opened well, to take loperamide so as to reduce bowel activity for the rest of the day.

The bottom line is that it is OK to experiment. Trial and error may be the only way to find out what suits you best.

More fibre or less fibre?

I don't think it's possible to answer that – it is really a matter of experimenting until you find what's best for you. More fibre may push you into diarrhoea-predominant IBS, which may then be controllable with low doses of loperamide. Less fibre in your diet may resolve the diarrhoea component but push you towards constipation-predominant IBS.

Could a food allergy or intolerance be causing my problems?

That's possible, and you might like to keep a detailed food diary to see if there is any association between what you are eating and the state of your bowel.

Do the antispasmodic medications help in IBS-A?

Yes, these are definitely worth trying. The diarrhoea component may be a consequence of spasm or part of a prominent gastro-colic reflex. This is a normal reflex whereby when the stomach distends with food, the bowel becomes more active. It is often more active in people with IBS, who might find themselves having to open their bowels whenever they begin to eat. Antispasmodic medication taken before the meal can help. In this context mebeverine (Colofac), and dicycloverine (dicyclomine, Merbentyl or Kolanticon gel) may be particularly helpful.

I do a lot of travelling. Could that be why my bowels are all over the place?

Travel is a common cause of a disturbed bowel habit. Many factors conspire to disturb your 'norm'. Inevitably, there is less control over both the timing and the content of your diet while travelling. More caffeine and alcohol will increase bowel activity. Stress usually causes constipation but in some people will lead to diarrhoea. Circumstances may mean that you have to suppress your need to go to the toilet, increasing the tendency to constipation. Finally, exposure to viruses and bacteria that are new to you can cause travellers' diarrhoea.

Constipation is the most common problem while travelling. If you are worried about taking laxatives, try suppositories. They usually work within half an hour.

If you are worried by diarrhoea during the journey, take loperamide. You can always take laxatives later. It's more important to enjoy your trip.

CONCLUSION

Irritable bowel with an alternating pattern can be very difficult to treat, and you must be ready to experiment. You will probably have to choose which of your symptoms is most disturbing, accepting that treating the constipation may make the diarrhoea worse and vice versa. Obtaining a completely normal bowel habit may unfortunately be impossible, but there are many simple treatments to try that will give you some control over your bowel.

SUMMARY

- About a third of people with IBS have both diarrhoea and constipation.

- People's main problem with IBS can change over time from diarrhoea to constipation and vice versa. IBS-A may be a transition state between the two.

- People with IBS-A should experiment with different treatments.

- You may have to choose whether to treat for diarrhoea and live with constipation, or vice versa.

10 | Food allergy and intolerance

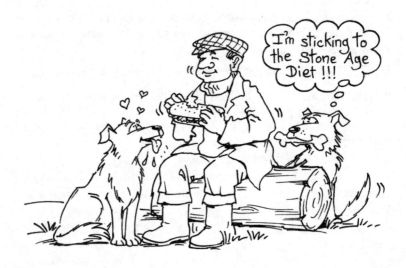

Many people are very willing to attribute all their digestive and irritable bowel problems to their diet. Sometimes they are right. But at other times, people can become totally obsessed with avoiding food that they think has previously upset them, refusing to accept continuing symptoms as evidence that their strategy has failed. If only someone would tell them what to eat and what not to eat, they feel all would be well. By contrast, doctors are mostly very sceptical about dietary interventions for irritable bowel, and they may show little interest in people's diet and offer little or no advice in this area. But both these extremes are unjustified. The purpose of this chapter is to describe how certain food allergies or intolerances can produce irritable bowel syndrome (IBS)-type symptoms, and which diets are worth trying.

Why are doctors sceptical about dietary interventions for IBS?

Doctors receive little training in nutrition and dietetics. They may see their role predominantly in terms of diagnosing and treating illnesses that have more ready cures. After diagnosing IBS, the only dietary intervention that some doctors know of is to increase the fibre intake. But more fibre only helps a minority of IBS patients, and the failure of this approach is taken as evidence against a dietary strategy. Moreover, patients readily tell their doctors of dietary changes that they have tried, and since people go to their doctors to report symptoms, the failure of their own dietary manipulations is taken as further proof that dietary interventions fail. Indeed, doctors can be very sceptical about anyone's ability to undertake any lifestyle change, however important it might be.

Finally, doctors like to use standard treatments that apply to most people with a given condition. This isn't just because it's easier and quicker to prescribe a treatment than to individualise it. By recommending 'standard' treatments, we get a feeling for how well they work and for the possible side effects. Otherwise it becomes more difficult to judge whether any apparent detrimental effect is a consequence of the treatment or of the condition being treated. With this knowledge, doctors can become very good at individualising drug-based treatments.

When it comes to dietary treatments, it becomes far more difficult. There is a lack of knowledge in general, as well as training, particularly among doctors. But more than that, there is a huge variability between people in their response to food. This means that there is no 'IBS diet'. If a dietary approach is to be successful, the diet needs to be individualised. This can be very time-consuming, and there is no guarantee of success.

What is the difference between a food allergy and a food intolerance?

Some people have unpleasant reactions to specific foods that most people find harmless. In an allergy, this adverse reaction is mediated by the immune system. In other words, the cells and antibodies designed to protect us against infection mistakenly target specific foods or components of foods. The symptoms are caused by the reaction of the immune system rather than by the food itself. A minute amount of food to which an individual is allergic can elicit a dramatic, even life-threatening, reaction. Chemicals secreted into the bloodstream by cells of the immune system are spread throughout the body, causing symptoms such as swelling of the face, difficulty breathing and a fall in blood pressure. The reaction can be severe enough for an individual to collapse to the floor, and may be life-threatening. Fortunately, such reactions are rare.

By contrast, a food intolerance does not involve the immune system. The adverse reaction to the food is caused by the direct chemical effect of the food or its components. Such reactions can be divided into three main groups. First is toxic or pharmacological. That is an expected reaction due to the known action of the food. For example, eating large amounts of rhubarb will cause loose stools in most people because rhubarb contains a natural laxative. Second, some people have a deficiency in their metabolism that leads them to react adversely to foods that are harmless to most people. Lactose or dairy food intolerance due to the absence of the enzyme lactase is an example of this (see more on this in Chapter 8). Third, some people react adversely to food, but the mechanism is unknown.

Does it matter if it's a food allergy or a food intolerance?

With a food allergy, the reaction can occur following a minute dose because it is amplified by the immune system. With a food intolerance, the extent of the reaction depends on the dose, so small amounts may be tolerated.

If my IBS is caused by a food allergy, does it matter for my long-term health if the allergy isn't identified?

Allergies that affect the respiratory system or cause facial swelling that may interfere with breathing can be life-threatening. People have died from nut allergies. But no one has died from IBS. As far as we know, food allergies and intolerances that produce IBS-type symptoms do not cause any long-term damage. The only exception to this is coeliac disease, which has been associated with an increased risk of cancer and osteoporosis if it goes untreated.

Last night my wife cooked cabbage mixed with bacon and spices. It was delicious, but in the night and today, I've had terrible pains in my lower abdomen. The pain has been coming and going in spasms, I've felt bloated, there has been a lot of noise from my tummy, and my stools have been loose. Do I have IBS, or am I intolerant of cabbage?

It may be neither. The most likely explanation is that your bowel is just reacting normally to a quantity of fibre or spice that it isn't used to. Fibre will bulk up your stool, holding water and gas in your bowel, and thus distending it. The spices may have stimulated more muscle activity. The result is bloating, spasm and loose stools. If you continue to eat this food, your bowel will probably adjust with time. For now, try smaller quantities.

I can understand how you could attribute your symptoms to the cabbage. My point is that the simpler explanation above is more likely. You may well have experienced similar symptoms in the past with other foods. If you attempt to avoid them all, your quality of life will suffer. Remember it may have been the quantity of cabbage that caused the problem, or it may have been the spices, or perhaps it was something else entirely.

COMMONLY IMPLICATED FOODS

Which foods are most commonly involved in food allergy?
And what symptoms do they cause?

Only eight foods or food groups (Table 10.1) are responsible for the vast majority of antibody-mediated food allergies. They mostly cause reactions affecting the entire body and are thus easily distinguished from IBS. In each case, antibodies called IgE antibodies are produced to react with a specific constituent of the food. The antibodies are present on the surface of specialised immune cells in the gut called mast cells. These cells make a variety of chemicals such as histamine that they store in granules within the cell. When an IgE antibody on a mast cell reacts with its specific food, the mast cell releases its granules. The chemicals released from the granules are then distributed in the bloodstream.

The reaction these chemicals produce often affects the whole body more than the gut. Swelling, especially of the face and lips, is caused by leakage of fluid from the blood vessels. The blood pressure falls because fluid has been lost from the circulation. Breathing can be difficult because of muscle spasm in the airways and fluid leakage into the lungs. In the skin, a localised leakage of fluid can cause an itchy rash called urticaria (hives). The gut responds with diarrhoea, vomiting, nausea and pain.

The severity of the reaction depends on how sensitive the individual is to the food and how much of the food has been taken. The reaction can be treated with antihistamines and adrenaline (epinephrine). In some cases, it can be prevented by a drug called sodium cromoglicate, which acts to stabilise mast cells and reduce their propensity to release their granules.

These food allergies are clearly nothing to do with IBS.

Table 10.1 The food groups causing antibody-mediated food allergy

Food group	Comment
Cows' milk	Up to 2% of infants are affected by this. Most become tolerant to cows' milk by 2 years of age
Eggs	This usually affects only infants and children, is usually mild and is usually outgrown
Fish	This mostly affects infants and children but has also been seen in adults
Wheat	Antibody-mediated wheat allergy is different from coeliac disease. It is usually mild and predominantly affects infants and children
Peanuts	The peanut is not a nut but a member of the legume family. Peanut allergy is claimed to affect up to 0.5% of the population. In contrast to other allergies that also begin in childhood, it is often not outgrown
Soyabeans	This is less common than peanut allergy. It can be outgrown, but it has been seen in adults
Crustaceans (shrimp, crab, lobster, crayfish)	In contrast to other allergies, this one seems to be more common in adults than children. It is also more common in Asia
Tree nuts (almond, hazel, walnut, brazil, cashew, pistachio, etc.)	Tree nut allergy may affect as many as 0.4% of the population. As with peanut allergy, it is not outgrown

Which foods are the most frequently implicated in IBS?

The most commonly incriminated foods are milk, eggs, nuts, wheat and fish.

Milk and dairy products

Milk is an important nutrient, providing almost half the calcium of the average British diet. It is also rich in vitamins and other minerals. Semi-skimmed milk is usually less than 2% fat. A daily glass of semi-skimmed milk provides a 6-year-old with all the vitamin B_{12}, around half of the calcium, phosphorus and vitamin B_2, about one third of the protein, potassium and iodine, and around one tenth of the vitamin A, vitamin B_1, niacin, vitamin B_6, folate, magnesium and zinc that he or she needs each day.

A few people are allergic to milk. More people may have lactose intolerance (see Chapter 8).

What's the difference between cows' milk allergy and lactose intolerance?

Cows' milk allergy is caused by an immune reaction to milk proteins. In lactose intolerance, there is no immune reaction; the symptoms are instead caused by a failure to digest lactose (the sugar in milk).

Cows' milk allergy occurs in up to 2% of infants, usually within the first 3 months of life. Some infants fed entirely on breast milk can become exquisitely sensitive to cows' milk, but in most the reaction is mild. The major symptoms are vomiting, diarrhoea and abdominal pain occurring within minutes to an hour of the milk being given.

In a few cases, the reaction is more serious, with facial swelling, wheezing and a fall in blood pressure. This is called anaphylaxis, and it occurs because immune cells in the gut carrying antibodies against the milk proteins have released large amounts of histamine and other chemicals into the bloodstream. These chemicals cause fluid to leak out of the blood vessels, causing swelling and a fall in blood pressure. At the same time, they can cause spasm of muscle in the airways of the lung, leading to wheezing and breathlessness. Fortunately, anaphylaxis is rare. The symptoms of cows' milk allergy become less severe with age, and most children are tolerant of milk products by 2 years of age.

Lactose intolerance occurs because most humans lose some of the ability to digest lactose in adulthood. Lactose is the sugar in dairy products. If it is undigested, it passes through the small bowel into the large bowel where, by holding water within the bowel, it causes diarrhoea. Some of the lactose is digested by bacteria to produce gas. The immune system is not involved, and the severity of the symptoms depends on the amount of lactose ingested. Most lactose-intolerant individuals can tolerate small amounts of lactose. Chapter 8 has more on lactose intolerance.

Wheat

Probably the most frequent dietary advice given to people with IBS is to increase the amount of fibre in their diet. They are exhorted to eat wholemeal bread, bran, wheat crackers and other high-fibre foods. Yet one of the foods most commonly reported as exacerbating IBS is wheat. This contradiction shows why people with IBS should take all dietary advice from non-dietitians with a pinch of salt.

I know that coeliac disease is related to wheat. Is coeliac disease a food allergy?

Yes, but in contrast to the food allergies described above, the immune reaction is not mediated by antibodies, but by cells localised to the small bowel. In coeliac disease, there is an abnormal immune response to gliadin, a constituent of wheat, rye and barley. This results in inflammation and damage to the lining of the small bowel. Symptoms arise because food cannot be properly digested and absorbed. Although antibodies to gliadin are present in the blood – and this is used as a screening test for coeliac disease – the antibodies are not involved in the disease process itself.

What is the difference between wheat intolerance and coeliac disease?

Some people with IBS feel much better on a wheat-free diet. When tested, they do not have coeliac disease, and other than provoking their IBS symptoms, wheat does them no harm. The mechanism behind this effect is unknown. It may be something in the wheat that they are unable to digest, or which bacteria in their bowel readily ferment to gas; or it may simply be that wheat-free diets include less fibre. In any case, it is reasonable to continue a wheat-free diet if your IBS responds to it, but the diet does not have to be strict or indefinite. By contrast, the gluten-free diet in coeliac disease has to continue indefinitely and be strict. Otherwise, the reaction to gliadin will recur and persist.

Lectins

What are lectins?

Lectins are naturally occurring plant proteins that are able to bind carbohydrate molecules. After they have been eaten and absorbed, the lectins can combine with carbohydrate molecules on the surface of cells, causing them to stick together. The damage can be extreme. For example, the poison ricin is a lectin derived from the castor bean, and as little as 500 µg can kill an adult.

Over 100 different lectins have been identified in foods, and it is tempting to speculate that they have some effect on our health and well-being. However, it is also possible that some plant lectins actually protect against some cancers, whereas others may cause disease. Some foods commonly implicated in IBS have been shown to contain lectins so this has made people interested in them in IBS.

So which foods contain lectins?

Lectins are present in plant foods, particularly in the peel. Table 10.2 gives a list (albeit an incomplete one) of common lectin-containing foods.

Does anything happen to lectins during cooking?

Most lectins in foods are deactivated and broken down by cooking. However, some lectins are remarkably heat resistant, including those of wheat, tomato, carrot, corn, rice, peanut and banana.

The increasing popularity of diets containing raw and relatively unprocessed foods probably means that some people are consuming more lectins now than at any time in human evolution. The 'stone-age diet' (see later in the chapter) is low in lectins, although it was not designed with lectins in mind.

Table 10.2 Foods containing lectins

Legumes	Grains	Vegetables	Fruits
Broad beans	Wheat	Avocados	Apples
Castor (oil) beans	Corn	Carrots	Bananas
Chickpeas	Rice	Mushrooms	
Green peas		Potatoes	
Lentils		Tomatoes	
Peanuts			
Red kidney beans			
Runner beans			
Soya beans			

Do lectins contribute to IBS?

Some people with IBS are much better when they avoid raw vegetables and fruit, or wheat. It is tempting to suppose that this improvement is a consequence of ingesting fewer lectins, but at present this is merely a guess.

Other food constituents that can have effects contributing to IBS

What does dietary fibre do?

Dietary fibre is indigestible plant carbohydrate (primarily cellulose pectins and lignins from the plant cell wall). It passes through the small bowel undigested to the large bowel, where bacteria partially metabolise it into gas, fluid and short-chain fatty acids. The short-chain fatty acids are absorbed by the large bowel and form an important nutrient. Most of the rest passes through in the stool along with water and gas trapped within it, and the bacteria living on it. Fibre therefore produces a softer, wetter, bulkier stool that is easier to pass.

Whenever I eat anything with a high fibre content, I get diarrhoea. Could I be intolerant or allergic to fibre?

You can call it an intolerance if you like, but actually looser stools are a natural consequence of eating more fibre, so there's nothing wrong.

What's the effect of caffeine?

Caffeine is a constituent of coffee, tea, cola and chocolate. It's thought to act by competing with the compound adenosine for its receptor on the cell walls. Adenosine is continually present in small amounts in the fluid surrounding all the cells in the body. It

Table 10.3 The effects of caffeine

	Physiological effects	Possible adverse effects with high doses in susceptible individuals
Brain	Stimulation Decreased fatigue Elevated mood	Agitation and nervousness Depression
Heart and circulation	Increased heart rate Higher blood pressure	Abnormal heart rhythms Angina High blood pressure
Gastrointestinal system	Increased acid production Decreased pressure in the lower oesophageal sphincter, the muscle that stops the stomach contents regurgitating Increased water and salt secretion by the bowel Increased bowel muscle activity	Dyspepsia (indigestion) Diarrhoea
Kidney	More urine being produced (diuresis)	Mild dehydration

reacts with a receptor on the cell surface and acts to 'dampen down' cell activity. By competing with adenosine, caffeine acts as a stimulant throughout the body, producing a multitude of effects to a greater or lesser extent in different people (Table 10.3).

Caffeine is a drug of addiction. Withdrawal symptoms include irritability, fatigue and headache.

What is the effect of salt?

In the long term, excess salt in the diet may contribute to cardiovascular disease. However, eating a meal with much more salt than you are used to can cause more immediate symptoms such as headache, thirst and bloating. These symptoms are probably due to fluid shifts within the body, initially from the bloodstream into the gut, and then from the rest of the body into the bloodstream.

Salt is sodium chloride, and it's the sodium that is the active component. In a Chinese meal, large amounts of sodium can be eaten as monosodium glutamate. It is therefore not uncommon to feel thirsty and bloated after a Chinese take-away.

What is monosodium glutamate, and what effects does it have?

Monosodium glutamate is the sodium salt of glutamic acid. Glutamate is a naturally occurring amino acid (a basic building block of protein) that is found in nearly all foods, especially high-protein foods such as dairy products, meat and fish, and in many vegetables. Foods often used for their flavouring properties, such as mushrooms and tomatoes, have high levels of naturally occurring glutamate.

Monosodium glutamate added to foods has a flavouring function similar to the glutamate that occurs naturally in foods. It acts as a flavour enhancer and adds a fifth taste, called 'umami', which is best described as a savoury, broth-like or meaty taste. In the European Union, monosodium glutamate is classified as a food additive (E621), and regulations are in place to determine how and when it can be added to foods. Typically, monosodium glutamate is added to savoury prepared and processed foods such as frozen foods, spice mixes, canned and dry soups, salad dressings and meat- or fish-based products. In some countries, it is used as a table-top seasoning.

Some people are sensitive to monosodium glutamate and suffer from what has been termed the 'Chinese restaurant syndrome'. About 10–20 minutes after a meal containing monosodium glutamate, they develop chest pain, flushing of the face and headache. The mechanism behind this reaction is unknown. The chest pain is not due to heart disease but is more likely to be caused by spasm in the oesophagus. Although this reaction has been associated with food containing large amounts of monosodium glutamate, such as Chinese food, the monosodium glutamate itself may not always be to blame as such foods also contain histamine, which produces similar reactions in the body during allergic reactions.

If histamine may be a culprit, which foods contain large amounts of histamine?

Histamine is one of the compounds released during an allergic reaction. It can have effects throughout the body that depend on where and how much histamine has been released. In a food allergy, histamine may be released from mast cells in the gut.

Interestingly, however, some foods can contain significant amounts of histamine, which can then be absorbed from the gut. If you have enough of them, a typical histamine reaction can occur, mimicking an allergic reaction. The symptoms may include urticaria (an itchy raised transient rash, also called hives), gastrointestinal symptoms such as abdominal pain, diarrhoea, nausea and vomiting, and facial flushing. Why some people are affected and others not probably relates to the variation in our ability to break down histamine before it is absorbed, and after it has been absorbed when it passes through the liver. The effects of histamine can be prevented by antihistamine tablets, which can be purchased over the counter.

Foods containing considerable amounts of histamine are yeast extracts, fish, chocolate, alcoholic drinks, and fermented products such as cheese, soy products, sauerkraut and processed meat. Histamine is produced in food by bacteria and yeasts. As a result, food that is overripe or decaying, especially fish and meat, may have very high quantities of histamine. Marmite has a particularly high concentration of histamine.

Scromboid poisoning is a severe reaction occurring 5 minutes to an hour after eating food containing large amounts of histamine, usually rotting tuna or mackerel. Symptoms are flushing, headache, dizziness, burning of the mouth and throat, nausea, vomiting, diarrhoea and palpitations.

What is the effect of spicy foods?

The typical effect of eating a highly spiced meal is an immediate feeling of fullness that can last for hours or even through to the next day. This may be because highly spiced food moves through the small intestine more slowly, as one study has shown. In spite of this, 60% of the people studied experienced mild diarrhoea, implying that spicy foods had opposite effects on the small and large intestines. Slowing down of the small intestine leads to bloating, while speeding up of the large bowel means that its contents are expelled as diarrhoea. There is currently no explanation for the effects of spicy foods on the gut. Many people with IBS find that their symptoms are exacerbated and take care to avoid spicy meals.

What is the effect of alcohol?

Alcohol can certainly cause and exacerbate gastrointestinal symptoms. It is a common cause of heartburn and other indigestion pains as well as diarrhoea. It is also possible that an individual is sensitive to the food from which the alcohol was derived rather than the alcohol itself. Interestingly, alcohol may also amplify the food intolerance response. So a meal containing wheat, for example, may only cause a problem if it is accompanied by alcohol. This can cause confusion when testing foods, but it may also be readily apparent from a food diary.

What about meat?

Meat, especially beef, gained a bad reputation for health when diets high in animal fat were associated with an increased risk of cardiovascular disease, strokes and heart attacks. But when trimmed of visible fat, beef is actually usually less than 10% fat. It is also an excellent source of protein, iron, zinc and the B vitamins. When it comes to food allergy, meat barely gets a mention; compared with other foods, meat intolerance is uncommon.

Meat contains virtually no fibre. Consequently, if you have constipation-predominant IBS, a diet high in meat may make you worse. Conversely, people with diarrhoea-predominant IBS may do better with more meat and fewer vegetables.

What about a vegetarian diet?

The vegetarian diet is inevitably high in fibre. So bloating, wind and diarrhoea will tend to be worse.

A DIETARY APPROACH TO IBS

What is an elimination diet?

An elimination diet is one in which specific foods or groups of foods are totally avoided. If a person's symptoms are due to specific food allergy or intolerance, avoiding that particular food should resolve the symptoms within 4–7 days. Reintroducing the food will lead to a recurrence of the symptoms, confirming the diagnosis. Elimination diets can therefore be used to diagnose and treat food allergies and intolerances. But in practice it isn't as easy as that.

When is it worth trying an elimination diet?

Food allergies and intolerances generally do not cause constipation, so it's only worth considering an elimination diet if diarrhoea is a predominant symptom.

How do you decide on which food to avoid?

There are a number of possible approaches.

1. You can avoid specific foods because you have associated them with symptoms. Keep a detailed food diary to guide you in choosing which foods to avoid.

2. You can avoid a few certain foods because they are known to commonly cause symptoms.

3. You can try a very restricted diet designed to be free of the more commonly non-tolerated foods. Once the symptoms have resolved, other foods can be reintroduced (called a food challenge) in the hope of identifying which specific food or foods are responsible for the symptoms.

How does a food diary help?

A diary detailing food consumed, along with any symptoms, may show which foods are associated with which symptoms, guiding you in your choice of foods to eliminate from your diet. It may also show that there is no connection between your diet and your symptoms. Ideally, you should detail all food and drink consumed, bowel movements, mood, stressful events, medications, exercise and

Figure 10.1 A simple food diary (one sheet per day).

Time	Food or drink	Symptoms

A more sophisticated food diary.

Time	Food or drink	Quantity and brand name	Symptoms	Bowel movements	Mood or social setting

symptoms. But even a simple list of just food and drink may be better than relying on memory.

You should keep a detailed food diary for at least 5 days, including a weekend, and ideally for longer. A simple food diary can be a few sheets of paper or a notebook. You can then extra add columns for any information that you feel is relevant. Examples are shown in Figure 10.1.

I've tried to avoid foods that seem to be associated with my symptoms, but my symptoms keep recurring. What can I do?

Most people approaching a physician or dietitian for help will already have tried to avoid foods that they believe are associated with their symptoms. Even if they are still avoiding certain foods, the strategy has failed to completely resolve their problem.

There may be a number of possible explanations for this failure. First, we all eat mixed meals, so it's very difficult to know which specific ingredient caused the problem. You may have eliminated the wrong food. A detailed food and symptom diary may suggest which foods to try avoiding.

Second, the food to be avoided may be widely used in the food industry and may thus be inadvertently ingested. Eggs, wheat and milk are examples of foods to which people are frequently intolerant or allergic but which are used in a huge range of products and may not be included in the ingredient list. For example, egg white or milk is used in clarifying wine.

Third, not all the foods causing the problem have been eliminated. And finally, the problem may not actually be a food allergy or intolerance.

I've got diarrhoea-predominant IBS. Which foods or groups of foods is it worth trying to avoid?

There are several relatively straightforward dietary manipulations that are worth trying.

A **lactose-free diet**. Avoid dairy products, including milk, butter, cheese and yoghurt. If you have lactose intolerance, there should be a dramatic improvement within a week. You can then reintroduce lactose to confirm the diagnosis. Even if the diagnosis is confirmed by re-testing, you may still be able tolerate small amounts of dairy products – yoghurt and hard cheese contain relatively little lactose. In addition, lactose tolerance may return in time so it's worth re-testing every few weeks or months.

A **fructose- and/or sorbitol-free diet**. These sugars can be difficult to digest, and diarrhoea occurs in some people if they are ingested in large quantities. Foods containing significant quantities of fructose are listed in Table 10.4.

Sorbitol, a polyol (a sugar alcohol), is a bulk sweetener found in numerous food products, including sugar-free sweets, chewing gums, frozen desserts and baked goods. It is also used as a base for medical products. Sorbitol is about 60% as sweet as sucrose with one third fewer calories. It has a sweet, cool and pleasant taste. Sorbitol is slowly converted to fructose in the intestine and may be poorly absorbed.

Sorbitol is known to cause diarrhoea in doses of more than 50 g a day. But some people may be more sensitive and suffer from diarrhoea and bloating at far smaller daily doses. Unfortunately, food labels may not state the quantity of sorbitol contained. In fact, despite the inclusion of sorbitol, the label may state that there is no added sugar. A sugar-free chewing gum probably contains 1 g of sorbitol per stick

Table 10.4 Fructose in food

Food	Fructose content (g per 100 g serving)
Chocolate	42
Honey	41
Dates	20
Pears	6
Cola drinks	6
Apples	6
Nectarines	5
Cherries	5

of gum, and some ice creams may contain much more. If you eat a significant quantity of 'sugar-free' products, it is very easy to ingest a sufficient quantity of sorbitol to produce diarrhoea.

A caffeine-free diet. A high intake of caffeine not only stimulates the gut but may increase nervous tension that could increase gut irritability.

A wheat-free diet. Some people with IBS, especially those in whom diarrhoea and bloating are the main symptoms, feel better on a wheat-free diet even if they do not have coeliac disease. We do not know why this should be, but there are several possibilities. Wheat fibre is one of the more laxative types of dietary fibre, so it is hardly surprising that eating less of it will improve diarrhoea-predominant problems. However, wheat may also be involved directly in food allergies, and it is in addition a source of dietary lectins (see earlier in the chapter).

An alcohol-free diet. A high intake of alcohol will certainly damage and irritate the gut, causing nausea, pain and diarrhoea. In severe cases, it can take 4 weeks of abstinence to resolve.

I haven't had any success with simple dietary manipulations. Now I want to try a more stringent elimination diet to see if this will improve my symptoms. What kinds of diet are available?

There are many suggested diets. Some possibilities are detailed in the tables and lists below. The rationale for such diets is twofold. First, trying to avoid particular foods can be difficult because many food products contain a mixture of ingredients. So diets that tell people what to eat rather than what not to eat are simpler to apply. Second, the more stringent the diet, the better the chance that the offending food or foods have been eliminated.

Once a symptom-free state has been established, it is possible to reintroduce foods one at a time (food challenge), with the aim of establishing which food or foods cause the problem.

The wheat-, milk- and egg-free diet

Wheat, milk and eggs are three common allergens that frequently come together in prepared food. So although it is possible to avoid one or other of these foods, some specialists recommend a diet that excludes all three.

Avoiding wheat

Foods with wheat may be labelled as containing any of the following: wheat grain, starch, flour, bran and farina. People with wheat intolerance or allergy should also avoid 'gluten-free' wheat starch as it is probably not the gluten to which they are reacting.

Baking powder, salad dressings, sausages, many gravies and many alcoholic drinks, including beer, lager and whisky, are also culprits. Even so-called 'pure' rye flour may contain wheat as the seeds are frequently contaminated. In any case, people who react to wheat are likely also to react to rye and barley.

Avoiding milk

Foods may be clearly labelled as containing milk or dairy products, but it should be noted that casein, caseinate, lactose and whey are also derived from milk. Even 'non-dairy' milk or cream substitutes may contain one of these derivatives. Many medicines contain some lactose as a base, as do artificial sweeteners.

Some foods should be assumed to contain milk or milk derivatives unless otherwise stated. These include non-dairy ice cream, chocolate and other sweets, margarine and bread.

Avoiding egg

Egg derivatives include vitellin, ovovitellin, livetine, ovomucin, ovomucoid and albumin. They are used in many common foods, including cakes, biscuits, bread, croissants, pastry, meringues, icing and sausages. Egg is also used in the production of wine, some instant coffee and root beer.

The stone-age diet

The stone-age diet looks back to an age before dairy products and grain became a staple part of our diet. Fossil evidence from groups of hunter-gatherers suggests that the daily diet was derived primarily from animal-based foods. In particular, our ancestors enjoyed animal organ meats like liver, kidney and brain – meat-foods that are extremely rich sources of nutrition. Stone-age humans did not consume much dairy food, nor did they eat high-carbohydrate foods such as legumes or yeast-containing foods, or cereal grains. It is said to be free of the more commonly non-tolerated foods and also contains fewer lectins.

Table 10.5 shows which foods are allowed in the stone-age diet. Foods not allowed are:

- cereal grains

- milk and all dairy products

- eggs

- potato

- soya

- tomato

- additives

- citrus fruits (orange, lemon, grapefruit, etc.).

- The diet can be changed if allergy or intolerance to one or other component is suspected.

The 'few-foods' diet

This diet provides a minimal set of foods thought to be the least likely to produce an allergic or intolerant response (Table 10.6).

Are there any problems with elimination diets?

Many people who may benefit from the diet initially suffer withdrawal effects over the first few days of the elimination diet. Headache is the most common symptom, but nausea, diarrhoea, fatigue, aching limbs, weakness, agitation and depression can also occur. Withdrawal symptoms are likely to be worse in people who were accustomed to drinking significant quantities of coffee and alcohol. Food cravings may also occur and may be severe. It is worth making a note of the craved-for food as it may subsequently prove to be responsible for the original symptoms.

Elimination diets are only for *short-term diagnostic use*. They are unlikely to be nutritionally adequate in the long term. Once the original symptoms have been resolved, foods are sequentially reintroduced to establish which food or foods are the cause of the problem.

Table 10.5 Foods allowed in the stone-age diet

	Food allowed
Fresh or frozen meat	Any kind
Fresh or frozen fish	Any kind
Fresh or frozen poultry	Any kind
Fresh vegetables	No potato, tomato or soya Any other kind (including sweet potato)
Fresh fruit	Any kind except citrus fruits
Grain	Rice, rice cakes, rice, noodles
Grain substitute	Buckwheat, quinoa
Drinks	Spring water, additive-free juices of allowed fruits, herb and fruit teas
Seasoning	Sea salt, fresh pepper, fresh herbs
Nuts	Allowed unless there is a known allergy
Oils	Olive oil, sunflower oil, safflower oil

Table 10.6 Foods allowed in the few-foods diet

Cod	Trout	Mackerel
Pears	Avocados	Swedes
Sweet potatoes	Quinoa	Beansprouts
Marrows	Courgettes	Cooked carrots
Safflower oil	Sea salt	Olive oil

How long should I continue an elimination diet before reintroducing foods?

If the original symptoms were occurring daily, you can begin to test foods as soon as they have cleared. Otherwise, you have to continue for sufficiently long to be sure that the symptoms have improved. If withdrawal symptoms occur, the diet should be continued until these have passed and there have been 2–3 days of freedom from symptoms.

How long should I try each newly introduced food for?

This depends on the symptoms you suspect have been caused by the food. Some reactions can occur within minutes. Others such as eczema or joint pains may take 2–3 days to appear. In general, gastrointestinal symptoms will take less than 8 hours to show up. In other words, if you suspect that milk gives you diarrhoea but don't have diarrhoea for 8 hours after drinking a pint of milk, you can conclude that the milk is innocent. You can continue to drink milk and try another food.

In general, one new food is reintroduced every fourth day, initially in small amounts, and then in normal servings on the next two days. If no reactions are observed for three consecutive days, the food can be included freely in the diet.

What if I still have symptoms despite a strict diet such as the stone-age diet or the few-foods diet?

It is possible that you are inadvertently still eating a food to which you are sensitive. But it is probably more likely that your symptoms are not caused by a food intolerance or allergy. The process of eating and digesting, the function of your gut, or the signalling process between your gut and your brain may be at fault, but the problem is not related to a specific food or foods.

How effective is the dietary approach as a treatment for IBS?

In some studies, almost half the people who complied with a highly restricted elimination diet responded. In other studies using similar methods, fewer than 1 in 6 people improved. Once the subjects had responded such that they had no, or minimal, symptoms, individual foods were reintroduced in order to identify the specific foods causing the symptoms. This is known as a food challenge. In general, people reporting diarrhoea were more frequently successful with this approach than were those with constipation.

How many foods are people with IBS usually intolerant to?

There is great variability between individuals. In those who are studied, about a third have between two and five food intolerances, about a third are intolerant to 6–10 foods, and a third are intolerant of more than 10 foods. Only about 1 in 20 are intolerant of just one food.

Can antibody testing help determine which foods to eliminate?

Possibly. In one study, the presence in the blood of an antibody called IgG antibody to various foods was determined for each individual participating. For each person, two diets were devised – one excluding all the foods to which the person had antibodies, and another, called the sham diet. The sham diet eliminated the same number of foods as the true diet, but these were foods to which there were no antibodies. The researchers tried to make the sham diet as difficult to follow as the true diet by eliminating the same number of staple foods in each diet. All the people participating had IBS. They were randomly allocated to follow a true or a sham diet, but they did not know which diet they were following. They continued the diet for 12 weeks and assessed the severity of their symptoms by completing a questionnaire.

The diets were difficult to follow, and almost a third of the participants in the study withdrew. But of those who continued the diet, either fully or partially, 28% improved on the true diet compared with 17% on the sham diet. About a third of individuals were able to adhere fully to the diet, and over half of these showed a significant improvement.

It is possible that testing for antibodies to food in the blood may be useful in determining which food to avoid. Such testing is not available on the NHS but is available commercially from Yorktest Laboratories (see the Appendix for details); it involves just a finger-prick blood sample.

Is there any alternative to an elimination diet for food allergy?

There is a drug called sodium cromoglicate that is thought to act by stabilising mast cells. These are the cells that react to the food allergen, releasing chemicals such as histamine, which cause the adverse reaction. Sodium cromoglicate is used in other allergic conditions such as asthma, and although it occasionally causes nausea, it is usually free of side effects and safe to take even in children. In one study, it was found to be as effective as an elimination diet, but this success has not been repeated. Unfortunately, sodium cromoglicate is not cheap – currently about £70 a month.

Are there any side effects from changing the diet?

Diets can affect our well-being. This is noticeable even to normal people when they eat a different diet on holiday. In the first few days, you can get withdrawal symptoms including irritability, fatigue and headache. Food cravings are common. Eating too little, especially eating too little carbohydrate, will result in ketone production from the fat stores. While this helps you to lose weight, ketones also cause nausea, headache, abdominal pain and fatigue.

If your new diet involves eating more fibre, then more bloating is almost inevitable in the first few days or even weeks. If your main problem is diarrhoea, more fibre may exacerbate it. Eating less fibre may help with bloating, but it may also contribute to constipation.

In the longer term, nutritional deficiencies are a worry. Iron deficiency is very common in vegetarians. People who avoid dairy products risk taking insufficient calcium in their diet. The longer we live, the more of a problem weak bones become.

Dieting can be socially restrictive and a terrible annoyance to the rest of the family. Keeping a detailed food diary, although possibly the most useful first step, can be enormously time-consuming, self-indulgent and the first step towards developing a food obsession. So if you keep one, keep it only until you have a result one way or the other.

CONCLUSION

A dietary approach to IBS may work for some people some of the time, but opinions differ on how effective it is and what to try first. It is more likely to work in diarrhoea-predominant IBS because constipation is unusual in food allergies and intolerances.

A dietary approach inevitably involves a lot of work, discipline and, most of all, experimentation. How much effort you wish to expend is your decision. Be aware of the huge variability between people, and be sceptical of 'miracle' diets. There is often variability for the same person too: what affects you today may not upset you tomorrow. This may be apparent from your food diary, and it implies that dietary manipulation will be unsuccessful. You may need to fall back on the famous saying by the American author Mark Twain, 'Part of the secret of success in life is to eat what you like and let the food fight it out inside.'

SUMMARY

- Food intolerance or allergy may be responsible for or exacerbate symptoms of IBS.

- People vary hugely in their response to specific foods.

- People vary over time. What may upset you today may not upset you tomorrow, and vice versa.

- Food allergies and intolerances generally do not cause constipation.

- People may be intolerant or allergic to multiple foods.

- Dietary interventions can be difficult and time-consuming, and there is no guarantee of success.

- An allergy involves the immune system, which amplifies the reaction, so a very small amount of the offending food can produce a severe effect.

- A food intolerance does not involve the immune system, and the effect of the offending food depends on how much of it is taken. Small amounts may be tolerated.

- The foods most commonly implicated in food allergy are cows' milk, eggs, fish, wheat, peanuts, soyabeans, crustaceans and nuts.

- The foods most commonly implicated in IBS are milk, eggs, wheat, nuts and fish.

- Caffeine, spicy foods and alcohol can all exacerbate the symptoms of IBS.

- Meat intolerance is uncommon.

- A food diary may show you whether there is an association between your diet and your symptoms, and suggest which foods you could try to avoid.

- If a person's symptoms are due to specific food allergy or intolerance, avoiding that particular food should resolve the symptoms within 4–7 days.

■ The most commonly attempted diets are the lactose-free diet and the wheat-free diet.

■ Beware of 'miracle' diets: there is no proven 'IBS diet'. Finding the right diet for you can involve a lot of hard work, diary-keeping, experimentation, discipline and luck!

■ Beware of avoiding so many foods that your diet becomes nutritionally inadequate. Seek professional advice from your doctor or dietitian.

■ As with any treatment, there is no guarantee of success, and there may be side effects.

11 | Psychological aspects of IBS

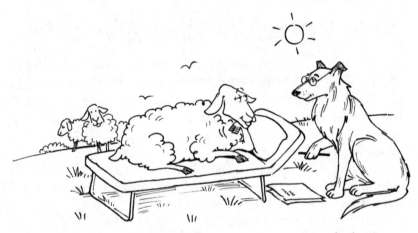

"Actually, I've never told anyone this before, but..."

WHY CONSIDER PSYCHOLOGICAL PROBLEMS?

I have IBS, a medical problem. Sure, I've had it a while, but why should I think about 'psychological problems'? I've got enough to deal with.

Dealing with irritable bowel syndrome (IBS) takes a lot of effort and is demanding. Anyone with IBS knows this and will admit that it can be emotionally stressful and draining. Did you know that about half of all people attending hospital clinics with IBS have an additional significant psychological problem such as anxiety or depression?

Psychological problems are probably no more common in people with IBS than in the general population. Nevertheless, most people with IBS will readily admit that their IBS symptoms are worse during times of psychological pressure. So there is a link between having IBS and a person's psychological state.

What sort of psychological symptoms are associated with IBS?

Many different psychological symptoms are associated with IBS. These are determined by the interaction between the individual's personality and the IBS. Some are common and occur in all shades of severity. These include anxiety, depression, loss of confidence, loneliness, secrecy and withdrawal, and acute embarrassment.

Remember that you're not alone. Psychological disorders are very common in the general population. Up to 1 in 4 women and 1 in 8 men will suffer from a major depression at some time in their life. Many more will have less severe mood disorders. And anxiety problems are even more common. Having any of these feelings does not mean that you have that disorder – feeling depressed, for example, does not mean that you therefore have a formal depressive illness.

Can anxiety cause gastrointestinal symptoms?

Gastrointestinal symptoms are very common in anxiety. The most common symptom is a dry mouth. Nausea and vomiting also occur and may be the dominant feature. The large bowel can also be disturbed, with diarrhoea or constipation. These symptoms occur due to activation of the autonomic nervous system (the automatic, unconscious part of the nervous system that controls the internal organs). They are usually associated with other physical manifestations of anxiety such as a cold sweat, a tremor and palpitations.

Do you think I'm a hypochondriac?

It is normal to worry about illness from time to time. Some people worry more than others, and they then worry that they will be seen as a hypochondriac. A short-lasting preoccupation with the fear of having a disease is fairly common. It usually occurs following a major life event, or when a person has experience of death or disease in a family member or friend. It is said to occur in over 70% of medical students at some time in their training!

What do doctors mean by the term 'hypochondriasis'?

In hypochondriasis, the fear of disease persists for months and years. People with this condition focus on thoughts about having a disease and constantly seek medical attention, but fail to be reassured by negative findings. Although fearful of disease, they rarely follow advice for a healthy lifestyle. They are more concerned with convincing the doctor that their illness is genuine. Unlike people with a serious illness, and most of those with IBS, people with hypochondriasis utterly reject any suggestion of an emotional element to their illness.

Do you think I'm depressed?

Depression is so common, either as a primary problem or as a consequence of other problems, that it should always be considered.

Most people know when they are depressed. They recognise that they are sad and acknowledge that this sadness is out of proportion to their situation. They may recognise irritability, frustration, worry, loss of libido, insomnia and fatigue as part of their depression. Gastrointestinal symptoms are also common and include loss of appetite, weight loss and an alteration in bowel habit. Sometimes these physical complaints come to predominate. People may not recognise them as part of a depression, or may attribute the depression to the physical symptoms. There is then a fruitless quest for a physical cause, which serves only to exacerbate the worry and frustration.

How can I tell if my abdominal symptoms are due to depression, or if I'm just frustrated by my continuing symptoms?

Depression is usually worse in the morning and lifts towards evening. It usually disturbs sleep with insomnia and early morning wakening, but it can occasionally cause excess sleep and sleepiness. By contrast, IBS rarely disturbs sleep even though many IBS patients complain of fatigue. It is not known whether fatigue in IBS is part of the syndrome or part of an associated depression.

People who are depressed often lose or gain weight. Surprisingly, despite the physical symptoms, weight is usually stable in IBS.

You should consider talking to your partner, friends or close colleagues. They may have noticed changes in your mood and behaviour that were not obvious to you.

Often, you can't be sure whether you are depressed, frustrated or both. Indeed, it may not really matter. If there is a significant depressive element to your illness, you should consider treatment. It is sometimes worth trying antidepressants even on just a suspicion of depression.

STRESS

What is stress?

The everyday experience of stress is easily identifiable and occurs when you have too much to do and too little time or money to do what is actually required. Essentially, the demands on you outstrip your internal supply of resources. IBS can be worsened by stress and can contribute to a stressful situation. The manifestations of stress can therefore be noticed in physical, behavioural and cognitive (thought) terms.

What are the physical effects of stress?

In physical terms, stress involves the co-ordinated response of the nervous system and the endocrine (hormone-secreting) system to prepare the body for unusually extreme activity. This has been termed the 'fight or flight' response.

The heart rate speeds up to deliver more blood to the muscles, breathing becomes faster to obtain more oxygen, and blood is diverted away from the gut, the kidneys and the skin to favour the muscles. The nervous system slows the gut down. Hormones such as adrenaline and cortisol (a steroid) are released and serve to stimulate the muscles and arouse the brain. The body gears itself up to run, fight or think rather than digest and excrete. In some people, the start of the stress response leads to an urge to defecate or pass urine.

Transient physical, emotional or psychological stress is perfectly normal and healthy. But stress that goes on for a prolonged period of time is thought to result in problems. The gut may be deluged with messages to slow down or speed up. The normal regulatory systems may be unable to make the fine adjustments necessary for normal function, and the gut may overreact to minor stimuli with severe reactions.

What are the behavioural effects of stress that may show up in IBS?

The behavioural response to stress and IBS may, for example, involve spending a lot of time getting to know the location of toilets, or avoiding going out altogether. Some people eat less; some people drink more alcohol. These responses may themselves cause yet more stress, leading to a vicious circle of stress–behavioural change–more stress, which ultimately depletes the person's resources until something has to give.

What is the cognitive response to stress in IBS?

The word 'cognitive' refers to the thoughts, beliefs and attitudes that colour our emotions and behaviour. For example, needing to use the bathroom in the middle of an important meeting can be awkward for most people. How you think about this situation can make all the difference. You could, for example, see the trip to bathroom as a chance for a break, or a rethink, and come back to the meeting re-energised.

Unfortunately, many people with IBS will be thinking negatively about themselves – 'My bowel is letting me down again, Why can't I hold on?', for example. What is worse is going on to assume that the other people at the meeting will also interpret your bathroom break negatively. It can destroy your confidence and exacerbate your stress if you feel that other people will think there is something wrong with you, that you can't handle the situation, that you're a failure, and so on.

This is how the cognitive response to an IBS problem increases a person's misery. And it is one area in which psychological therapy can help. You may not be able to control your need to visit the bathroom, but you can learn to understand and control your cognitive response.

What's the relationship between emotional feelings and the physical aspects of IBS?

It's essentially a vicious circle. The original cause of the IBS may be a mixture of physical and psychological factors. In some people, emotional problems can be transformed in the mind into physical symptoms because that is the safest way of dealing with them. The IBS then becomes a useful 'final common pathway' for both factors, physical and psychological.

But having IBS is a stressful experience and can lead to very powerful feelings and other psychological problems. These experiences may be felt directly or may themselves be transformed into physical conditions and then become part of the IBS. For example, the IBS may be in part caused by depression, but it is also a depressing condition to have.

PSYCHOLOGICAL TREATMENT

The primary cause of IBS may not be a psychological illness. But there is often an important psychological element that exacerbates and prolongs the problems and makes the symptoms more difficult to deal with. The treatment approaches to these psychological elements differ in terms of how far they call upon the individual to be engaged in the treatment and the psychological 'depth' that is potentially reached. Treatments that can be less demanding on the person include informal discussion with the family doctor and the use of medication. Those requiring more involvement are well described by cognitive behavioural therapy and psychoanalytic psychotherapy.

What do you mean by 'informal psychological treatment'?

'Informal psychological treatment' occurs whenever you discuss your problems with someone. The process of putting the problems into words and expressing them to other people may give you a better sense of perspective on the situation and make you feel less burdened. Talking with your doctor will hopefully bring more authoritative reassurance, along with education and perhaps some useful ideas and possible other treatments. Many doctors will use some of the cognitive and behavioural techniques described below, without calling them this, as part of their normal consultation.

What aspects of a consultation with the doctor are psychologically helpful?

Allowing people to describe in detail what for them may be very embarrassing problems is the first part of a successful consultation. This is followed by the reassurance from someone who knows.

Part of the reassurance involves 'making a diagnosis', giving the disease a name and so 'legitimising' the symptoms.

But what if the doctor can't give a reassuring diagnosis?

It may not be possible at the first consultation for the doctor to be completely reassuring. For example, a test may be required to check for cancer. Some people will immediately think that there is a cancer there and will go on to imagine the very worst. In this situation, it can be useful for the doctor to be completely up front with the possible diagnosis rather than to offer bland reassurance that will not be believed. People may respond better to a simple statement of facts, for example, 'Yes, we are going to perform a colonoscopy to check for cancer, but the chance of finding it is only about 1 in 10.'

Some people will insist on thinking the worst. For them, describing the worst-case scenario may help as what they would otherwise imagine is invariably worse. There are other people who really do not want to know. This can be a conscious or unconscious decision. It is a kind of pretending that there is nothing wrong; this is called 'denial'. It can be a useful psychological protection mechanism, and most of the time it turns out that there was nothing at all to worry about. To my mind, 'denial' should be respected by the doctor as far as possible. Unfortunately, the current emphasis by the medical regulatory authorities and lawyers on fully 'informed consent' for procedures sometimes makes this difficult and can lead to unnecessary anxiety.

Can the doctor–patient consultation for IBS go wrong?

Even the most experienced, sympathetic and knowledgeable doctor will have an unsuccessful consultation from time to time in which both parties will come away feeling unhappy. Discussions about diseases that have no clear cause or solution take considerably more time than those dealing with usually 'simple' problems such as stomach ulcers. Appointment systems cannot cater for this discrepancy, especially as on many occasions the diagnosis isn't known when the appointment is booked.

People find it helpful to talk about their symptoms in detail and at length, but doctors often diagnose by pattern recognition and 'know' the diagnosis early on in the consultation. The doctor will want to ask specific questions to confirm or deny this prospective diagnosis, but the person with the condition may want to go on talking about symptoms that the doctor now considers irrelevant. The doctor's priority is to look for serious disease; the individual may be confident that he or she has IBS and just want advice on symptom management. The doctor may feel that the problem is at least partly psychological; the person may feel that his or her physical symptoms are not being taken seriously. So the two of them can continue to annoy each other for the whole consultation.

These are just a few of the potential problems that can occur when going to see the doctor about IBS. If there were a really effective medical treatment for IBS, people would find it easier to forgive their doctors. Unfortunately, this is not yet the case.

WHAT ABOUT MEDICATION?

Antidepressant treatment is discussed in the chapter on pain (Chapter 4). It is one of the most useful treatments for IBS. Pain may be reduced even if there is no depression, and the improvement may occur with low doses within just a few days.

FORMAL PSYCHOLOGICAL TREATMENT

Cognitive behavioural therapy (CBT)

What is cognitive behavioural treatment?

This is a treatment provided by psychologists using cognitive (thinking) and behavioural (action) techniques. The cognitive approach assumes that how we think and interpret our experiences affects our emotions and general well-being. Thoughts come before feelings. In other words, having negative thoughts makes us feel worse, whereas positive thoughts can make us better.

The behavioural approach puts the emphasis on what we actually do rather than what we think or feel. Put simply, if we behave normally, we will be normal. If we behave like an invalid, we will be an invalid.

What does a case using CBT 'look like'?

Here's one. Mrs A was a very busy woman. It wasn't easy being a wife and mother as well as holding down a job. On top of all that, she also had IBS. Mrs A had never really been sure when it had developed, but it had become another aspect of her already busy life that she had had to manage. Her husband was supportive as long as it didn't interfere too much in their lives and as long as she kept the details about her IBS down to a minimum.

One day, while rushing around the shops, Mrs A suffered an attack of IBS. It was so bad and urgent that she very narrowly avoided having a major accident, but she found herself in the ladies toilet with soiled underwear and a faintly soiled skirt. She was really embarrassed and upset. She confided in her best friend and, after a heart-to-heart, her friend suggested that perhaps she should find some professional help.

Mrs A approached her family doctor, who referred her to the

clinical psychology service in her area. Mrs A went on to meet Miss T for a consultation, and they agreed to an initial contract of 12 hour-long sessions.

Mrs A initially needed to keep a detailed diary of her daily activities, her bowel motions, her experience with her IBS symptoms, what she thought when these occurred and how she felt during every day. In her meetings with Miss T, the two of them would discuss the diary entries to a level of detail that surprised Mrs A, but it was an aspect of the treatment that she quickly embraced.

This approach was very enlightening for Mrs A. She realised that she expected herself to pass a stool at the beginning of every day and that the stool had to clear her bowel entirely. If these two beliefs were not confirmed by events, Mrs A tended to think that she would then have an attack of IBS, so she felt pressured, lacked confidence and restricted going out so that she only went to places where she had easy access to a toilet. So, in her morning routine, Mrs A sat on the toilet straining for long periods to try and prevent all this happening.

Miss T was able to help Mrs A challenge her own thoughts and try and find evidence to back them up. Encouraged, Mrs A found out that it was not necessary to empty her bowel every day. She learned that the feeling of an incomplete motion was very common in IBS and did not signify an ongoing attack. She did not therefore need to strain on the toilet. More importantly, by examining and talking about the evidence in her diary, Mrs A was able to identify what pattern of bowel motion was normal for her and therefore begin to plan her working day and movements to accommodate this.

As the sessions progressed, Mrs A became increasingly able to notice how thoughts that were self-deprecating often flashed through her mind. She learnt how to identify these and then ask herself for evidence of whether or not these were correct. Her confidence and sense of control increased. As a result, whether an episode of IBS occurred or not had less devastating consequences for her.

Interestingly, in the course of the 12 sessions, Miss T noted how Mrs A would often make huge, overwhelming conclusions based on very meagre evidence. On the first occasion, Mrs A seemed to conclude that she had cancer because she felt pain that kept coming back and did not seem to be helped by any treatment. As a result, she felt extremely anxious for long periods of time. Miss T helped Mrs A to evaluate the evidence that was available, such as the length of time she had felt the pain, which was in fact several years, the intermittent nature of the pain, which did not suggest a problem there all the time, the absence of other factors such as weight loss, and the length of time that Mrs A had thought she had had cancer. Given all this, if Mrs A did have cancer, she should have been dead by then.

This was all a bit of a revelation to Mrs A, who then understood that she had a tendency to come to the most catastrophic conclusions on the basis of very little evidence. She thought that this might have been linked to her experience of seeing her mother do the same, but there seemed too little time in the contract with Miss T to explore this further.

By the end of her sessions, Mrs A had learnt how to make careful observations of herself and her thoughts and to challenge those which she felt were automatic and negative. For example, in the morning she would catch herself thinking, 'Oh dear, what a disappointing poo. I'm really going to have a bad day today' – an automatic thought (see more on this later). Previously, this thought would not only have made her depressed and anxious, but might also even have curtailed her planned activities.

Now Mrs A had learned to question this thought by asking herself what actual evidence she had that the quality of her poo was the major determinant of the quality of her day, and to challenge this thought by purposely remembering good days that had occurred despite a 'disappointing poo'. She gained much more control of her IBS, and this appeared to lead to an overall increase in confidence in other aspects of her life. Mrs A occasionally had a bad day, but in that case she applied her method of assessing the evidence, and this undoubtedly helped her. Soon this method became automatic, and Mrs A could not imagine how she could have been so dominated by her IBS before.

Put simply, what are the core ideas underlying a cognitive behavioural approach?

CBT had its origins in a treatment for depression, but it has quickly become established as a powerful, relatively short-term treatment method for a variety of problems. It assumes that behaviour is brought about by the individual's thoughts, and that feelings are a result of these thoughts. There are different classes of thought and belief, from those which flash through the person's mind without them noticing, to those which are so deep-rooted that they form the basis of a person's basic identity. Most of these thoughts are outside awareness, and they develop as a result of life experience.

Psychological difficulties arise when the thoughts that flash through the mind are essentially negative and detrimental to the person themselves. These 'negative automatic thoughts' are never challenged but dictate an individual's response and therefore mood. The negative automatic thoughts are in turn based on more deeply rooted assumptions that are themselves wrong. These are therefore termed 'dysfunctional assumptions'.

CBT aims to teach individuals to notice and then challenge their own thoughts. Clients and therapists are seen as partners in this to work out exactly what is going on in the clients' mind whenever they feel unwell and unhappy. Once identified, these thoughts need to be assessed on the basis of the available evidence and must then stand or fall. Becoming good at this is the key skill in CBT, and after a while it becomes possible to generalise across automatic thoughts and begin to identify the assumptions that these are based on.

Gradually, the individual is helped to regain control over his or her own mind in relation to the specific problem. It is not difficult therefore to understand that CBT usually works best with a well-defined difficulty rather than a sense of general malaise. Focusing on symptoms in this way may initially cause them to get worse, but they should improve as the therapy develops.

Overall, a course of CBT usually involves about 12 sessions, each lasting 50–90 minutes. Each session involves feedback from the previous session, a review of 'homework', identifying cognitive and behavioural factors that are maintaining the IBS, devising strategies to cope with and minimise those factors, setting goals and agreeing on the next homework.

Psychodynamic psychotherapy/psychoanalysis

What does psychodynamic psychotherapy/psychoanalysis 'look like'?

Mr B had had IBS for many years and managed fairly well. He had a good relationship with his doctor and had adopted a live-and-let-live attitude towards his IBS. He tolerated it and in return felt that it behaved itself and did not attack him too vigorously. He had worked all his life, was reliable and loved his wife and children. Like everyone else, he had had his fair share of disappointments, such as not being promoted at work as high as he felt he should have been, but he felt that these were more than made up for by the overall balance of his life.

One day, Mr B had an attack of IBS. At first, he was not overly concerned. It had happened before and would no doubt happen again. He would just have to ride it out and manage in the way he had always done. But this attack was different. It didn't really stop, even though it lessened somewhat, and Mr B never felt settled. It would occasionally even get worse suddenly. It just went on and on, and Mr B couldn't understand why it had happened and why it wouldn't stop.

After a while, it became really tiring and wore down Mr B's patience and energy. Exasperated, he spoke to his GP, who then referred him to his consultant for an expert opinion. Mr B met with his consultant, and together they reviewed his case. Nothing appeared to have changed, and additional investigations did not produce any significant findings. His consultant then suggested that Mr B meet a colleague of his, Dr H, who was a psychoanalytic psychotherapist. Mr B had never thought of visiting a 'quack' but thought he had nothing to lose; anyway, he did not want to disappoint his consultant, who had helped him so much in the past and whose recent efforts he really appreciated.

So Mr B met Dr H for an initial consultation. He found Dr H rather easy to talk to, and although he was a bit nervous, he agreed to come and see Dr H for a 50-minute chat three times a week. Dr H had initially suggested to Mr B that they meet five times a week, but Mr B did not feel he either wanted this or could afford the time or money for it.

Initially, Mr B found great relief in meeting Dr H. Yes, it was strange that Dr H never mentioned anything about his own personal life and insisted on beginning and ending the sessions at the times they had initially agreed. It was also a bit strange to lie down on a couch and not actually be able to see Dr H, but Mr B found that after a while it was quite pleasant. After all, he could say exactly what came to his mind and not have to pay attention to Dr H all the time! This made him feel a bit better, and Mr B found that he could tell Dr H about his experience of IBS.

Together, they realised that the current attack of IBS had begun shortly after Mr B had learnt that an ambitious ex-trainee of his had been promoted over him and could now theoretically tell Mr B what to do. Additionally, and as their relationship grew, Mr B increasingly told Dr H about his past and how he had always to be careful not to upset his father, whose job often took him away from home, while at the same time he had missed his father very much.

But unfortunately, Mr B's IBS did not seem to improve greatly, and as much as he liked Dr H, this frustrated him. On top of this, Dr H always seemed to translate what Mr B said into some statement about Mr B himself. Some of these points were very interesting, but after a while it became a bit tiring. The final straw came when Mr B started arguing with his wife about the cost of his therapy. She felt that they could use the money in better ways, especially as the IBS didn't seem to be improving. Mr B suffered a really bad attack of IBS, was really angry with Dr H and felt that the therapy had come to an end.

To Mr B's surprise, though, Dr H talked to him about his dilemma in being angry and how this clashed with his valuing the time and effort that Dr H had given to Mr B. Dr H pointed out how Mr B could not believe that Dr H understood his anger while he simultaneously did not lose sight of the fact that Mr B valued their work together. It was as if Mr B felt his anger to be purely destructive, of no use and something to be got rid of. Mr B did not quite understand but he felt very relieved, and surprisingly his IBS attack resolved very quickly, staying that way for longer than Mr B expected. Over the next few weeks, he decided to stay with the therapy.

As their work subsequently proceeded, Mr B learnt that it was actually possible to be angry with Dr H without Dr H being destroyed by the anger or resentful of it. With more time and work, Mr B realised how afraid he had been of being angry and aggressive with his father as he had, in his mind, associated this with his father leaving home and Mr B feeling empty and bereft. Mr B had felt it too risky both to want his father but to be angry at him for his absence, because it seemed that in his mind such feelings had caused his father to leave rather than be there for Mr B. Anger, frustration and desire were a risky emotional mix, and it had seemed safer to expel all three from his mind.

Slowly, and by examining what had occurred in his relationship with Dr H, Mr B was able to allow himself to learn about his anxieties and resistances towards his own feelings of anger, frustration and desire, and feel them in an increasingly confident manner. He was also pleased that his IBS seemed to have got significantly better, and although he occasionally had a mild spell, he was far less concerned about it than he had ever been before. Indeed, Mr B became more dedicated to his job, felt much more respected by his peers and, to his great surprise, had a more alive and fulfilling relationship with his wife than he had ever expected.

After just under 4 years of therapy, Mr B and Dr H decided to end the treatment. Although Mr B knew he could always return to Dr H if he felt he wanted to, he was struck, as he walked out of the consulting room for the last time, by the fact that he still didn't know much about Dr H himself – but that it didn't really matter.

So, put simply, what are the core ideas underlying a psycho-analytic approach?

Psychoanalysis as a treatment started about 100 years ago and was originally developed by Sigmund Freud. Since then, it has expanded enormously and is still doing so. Central to the psychoanalytic model are the idea of the Unconscious, the importance of feelings and the notion of conflict. It is thought that experienced difficulties sometimes represent an acceptable way of expressing conflicts within the mind that are actually too risky to deal with consciously.

In the above example, the conflict in Mr B's mind involved love for his father versus anger towards his father. The conflict could not be resolved because Mr B's young mind had associated anger at his father with his father leaving home. He could not risk expressing anger for fear of loss. Difficulty expressing anger became a part of his personality, and this unexpressed emotion eventually manifested as physical symptoms, in his case as exacerbations of IBS. Mr B was unaware of these internal conflicts because they had developed and become embedded when he was a young child, long before he understood anything about thoughts and feelings.

Psychotherapists accept that the mind does not work just according to logic, so many people find themselves making the same sorts of mistake and/or having the same sort of difficulties over and over again. By entering a stable and consistent relationship with a properly trained psychotherapist, these underlying conflicts can gradually emerge in the relationship with the therapist and, as the therapist interprets them, can be more consciously worked on so that they might be resolved.

A crucial factor is how the client experiences the relationship with the therapist, which is why the psychotherapist will not divulge personal information. It is also why the times of sessions are fixed and not changed from week to week, even though the latter may seem more convenient. Finally, given the depth of the psychological work done, psychoanalytic psychotherapies tend to take much longer than other forms of treatment, although this in turn means that the benefits of psychotherapy are usually more widespread than only being focused on the original problem.

Do psychological treatments work, and what might be expected of me?

Modern research into all forms of psychological treatment is only about 55 years old at present. Evaluating psychological treatment programmes is notoriously difficult, and all the results need to be taken with a pinch of salt; unlike testing medicines, for example, psychological treatments cannot be tested in a what is called a double-blind manner, when neither the therapist nor the client knows who is receiving a real treatment and who is receiving a placebo (dummy treatment). With psychoanalysis, both the client and the therapist know what treatment is being given, and this knowledge may affect the result.

Studies looking at CBT in IBS have mostly been rather small, with fewer than 50 subjects. Despite this, there is agreement that CBT is as effective as, and possibly superior to, other psychological treatments as well as conventional medical therapy in IBS. In the largest study of CBT, over 400 patients were randomly allocated to receive CBT, an antidepressant (antidepressant treatments for IBS are discussed in Chapter 4), a placebo or education on their condition. The placebo (an inert, ineffective tablet) helped in 49% of individuals, which is a common finding in IBS studies. CBT was effective in 70% of subjects, and the antidepressant was effective in 60%. The usual criticism of studies like this is that they do not follow up their subjects for very long after the end of the treatment, so it is difficult to know whether these positive effects actually persisted.

There have only been a few studies on psychodynamic psychotherapy for IBS. All of them show it to be more successful than medical treatment alone or than 'sympathetic listening' from, for example, a nurse. The most recent and largest study, published in 2003, looked at 257 individuals with IBS and severe abdominal pain who had not responded to usual medical treatments over 3 months. These people were randomly allocated to receive psychotherapy or the antidepressant paroxetine (an SSRI type of antidepressant; see Chapter 4), or to continue the medical therapy they were already having. They were reassessed after 3 months and again after 5 months. Disappointingly, there was only a small improvement in the symptom scores from all three groups. No one treatment proved to be any better than any other.

Findings such as those above emphasise a general factor reported in research – that the more motivated the person, the better chance any therapy has of working. Psychological treatments involve a lot more effort than just taking a tablet or avoiding certain foods. People have to think about themselves and their problems in ways that they have not tried before. The approach may appear alien and incomprehensible at first and can be psychologically painful. Any psychological treatment requires an investment of time and effort, but most of all, people must be prepared to talk about their personal thoughts and feelings. Moreover, they must be prepared to have their assumptions about themselves challenged. The prize to be aimed for is better control of your life through self-knowledge and awareness.

OK, I want to try a psychological route to tackling my IBS. What now? Where do I go?

Unfortunately, psychology services are relatively poorly available in the UK, and CBT for IBS is not readily available in most hospitals. Furthermore, psychological services in the UK are not currently regulated by law, so although there are many well-trained therapists, there are also many very poor or untrained ones. Your family doctor is always a good place to start. Or, for properly qualified clinical psychologists who practise CBT, you could try the British Psychological Society. For psychoanalytic therapy, you should contact the London Clinic of Psychoanalysis. Both organisations are highly reputable (see the Appendix for contact details).

CONCLUSION

Most people with IBS will acknowledge that their symptoms are worse at times of stress or psychological difficulty. Which came first – the IBS or the psychological problem – is difficult to determine and probably does not matter anyway as it is clear that each will exacerbate the other. Just as it is worth trying the various physical therapies available, so it is worth exploring the psychological aspects of IBS. Admitting that you have some psychological areas to deal with does not mean denying your physical symptoms. It does not mean that 'it is all in the mind', that you are, for example, expected to stop your medication. It is just another way of getting control of your symptoms and of gaining the self-knowledge that may help in other aspects of your life.

SUMMARY

- Psychological disorders are very common in the general population.

- Gastrointestinal symptoms are very common in anxiety.

- Transient physical, emotional or psychological stress is perfectly normal and healthy. But stress that goes on for a prolonged period of time is thought to result in problems.

- IBS can cause psychological distress, and it may itself be caused or aggravated by psychological distress. Regardless of which came first, alleviating psychological distress is likely to help.

- Informal psychological treatment happens all the time, when talking to friends, relatives and healthcare professionals.

- The process of putting your problems into words and expressing them to other people may give you a better sense of perspective on the situation and make you feel less burdened.

■ CBT is a treatment provided by clinical psychologists using cognitive (thinking) and behavioural (action) techniques. Thoughts come before feelings. In other words, having negative thoughts makes us feel worse, whereas positive thoughts can make us better.

■ In psychodynamic psychotherapy, a trained psychotherapist listens to individual people talking about their innermost feelings. An intense relationship develops in the service of understanding how the person's emotional life interacts with his or her physical and psychological symptoms, and in thereby alleviating the distress caused.

■ Psychological treatments involve a major investment of time, money and emotion.

■ Take care that you are consulting a properly qualified psychologist.

■ The ultimate aim is a better life through self-knowledge and awareness.

12 | Complementary medicine

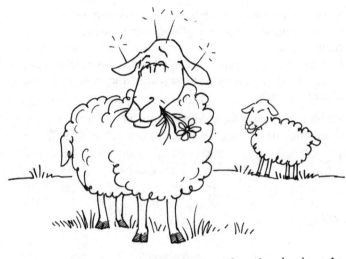

'Yes, very relaxing, but I prefer the herbs...'

'Complementary medicine' refers to a group of therapeutic and diagnostic disciplines that exist largely outside the places where conventional health care is provided and are not usually available on the NHS. These disciplines were previously known as 'alternative medicine', but their increasing use alongside conventional medicine has led to the term 'complementary medicine'. Unfortunately, this has only increased the considerable confusion over what exactly complementary medicine is, and what position the various disciplines included under this term should hold in relation to conventional medicine. Only a few of these disciplines are discussed in this chapter.

COMPLEMENTARY MEDICINE
AND THE PLACEBO RESPONSE

*My doctor tells me that his practice is 'evidence based'. He is
sceptical about complementary medicine and feels it is mostly a
placebo response. What is a placebo response?*

A placebo response is the measurable, observable or felt improvement in health that cannot be attributed to the treatment itself
but stems from a belief in, or indeed the process of, being treated. In
the placebo effect, the doctor's belief in the treatment and the individual's faith in the doctor are mutually reinforcing. The result is a
powerful remedy that is almost guaranteed to produce an improvement. This is very useful in clinical medical practice but makes it
difficult to determine how effective any treatment actually is.

How long does the placebo response last?

The placebo response has been shown to last up to 3 months.

How do we know if a treatment works?

The scientific method of evaluating treatments is designed to
reduce the effect of the placebo response. It usually involves what
is called a 'randomised double-blind placebo-controlled trial'. In one
of these, subjects are randomly allocated to receive either the treatment being tested or a sham, ineffective treatment – the placebo.
Both the true treatment and the placebo look exactly the same, and
people do not know which they are getting. That is what is meant by
being 'blinded' to the treatment, which is coded as, for example, 'X'
or 'Y'. In a double-blind study, the person assessing the success or
failure of the treatment also does not know which treatment the
'subject' has had, so cannot, either consciously or unconsciously,

influence the result. At the end of the study, the code is broken and the success of the two treatments can be compared.

In many medical conditions, the response to the placebo (sham or ineffective treatment) is surprisingly high. In irritable bowel syndrome (IBS), placebo response rates are usually between 30% and 50%, although they can be higher than this. In other words, many people are made better by treatments that are known to have absolutely no physical or biochemical effects. If a drug is to be regarded as effective in conventional medicine, it must prove itself consistently and significantly more effective than a placebo.

Can complementary medical treatments be tested using one of these double-blind placebo-controlled trials?

Some therapists claim that, for their treatments to be effective, they need to treat the person as a whole. This means altering the treatment to suit the individual. As this process involves a close interaction with the therapist, and the treatment has to be adjusted, it is difficult to give a placebo. It is also difficult for the individual and the therapist to be 'blinded' to the treatment, as described in the previous question. Furthermore, conventional medicines are tested by comparing a large group of people receiving one treatment with another large group receiving a different treatment or placebo. In complementary medicine, people with the same condition may end up receiving different individualised treatments, so it may not fit into the usual 'medical model' and cannot be tested in the conventional way.

Despite this, some complementary medicines, particularly some herbal remedies and Chinese medicines, have been tested in a few randomised double-blind placebo-controlled trials, sometimes with successful results.

Should I try complementary medicines for my IBS?

Compared with conventional medicines, complementary medicines are largely untested, and their effectiveness has yet to be proved. Their use is mostly limited to disorders that conventional medicine does not treat satisfactorily. For example, 30 years ago it would have been reasonable to try complementary medicine for peptic ulcers. But in 1976, cimetidine (Tagamet), the first drug specifically designed to reduce acid secretion became available. Today, conventional medicines for peptic ulcers are so effective and safe that if they fail to work, the diagnosis should be questioned. Cimetidine, and the drugs that followed in its wake, revolutionised the treatment of peptic ulcers. It would be stupid to use an alternative treatment for this condition.

Sadly, people with IBS are still waiting for the miracle cure. In IBS, conventional medicines can be disappointing, and if you can afford the expense, complementary alternatives may be worth trying; the placebo response itself may help you and shows the power that positive thought can have.

Sometimes people can feel pressurised to line up on one side or the other of the debate on conventional medicine. Although it may be contradictory to believe strongly in the scientific method while trying complementary medicines, holding on to contradictory belief systems – and acting on both – is very human. We suspend belief every day to enjoy novels and films. And, contrary to the evidence before us, many people believe in the eventual triumph of the England cricket and football teams! You never know what will work. Sometimes you just have to try as it may be right for you.

Have I got anything to lose by trying complementary medicine?

You need to be sure first that you do not have a condition that is more amenable to conventional medicine than IBS. Complementary medicine does not work for bowel cancer, and it's foolish to try for a placebo response or something better while delaying a conventional medical diagnosis and treatment. Similarly, complementary medicine has little to contribute to coeliac disease or inflammatory bowel disease (see Chapter 8). You also usually have to pay for complementary medicine, and the expense can soon mount up, so it's worth making sure that you've tried conventional treatments as well.

HERBAL MEDICINE

What are herbal medicines, and how do they differ from conventional medicines?

Many conventional drugs are based on herbal remedies or plants. The best known examples are aspirin, which comes from willow bark, and morphine, which comes from the opium poppy. Modern medicine and pharmacology have tried to isolate any active ingredient, purify it and modify it to make it more potent or to decrease its side effects.

By contrast, herbalists use unpurified plant extracts. Herbal preparations are likely to contain several active constituents, especially if several different herbs have been used together. Moreover, the constituents in two samples of a particular herbal drug may be in different proportions. Herbalists claim that combining several constituents reduces the toxicity of the whole treatment, a concept they call 'buffering', and that the interaction between the different herbs means that the treatment is more effective. Chinese herbs, for example, are selected and combined in formulas based on principles that have no relation to biochemistry. The vast majority of herbal treatments use formulas containing four or more herbs. By contrast, conventional practice tries to limit the number of drugs being taken whenever possible.

Do herbalists make a diagnosis?

Herbal practitioners take a history and may perform a physical examination. They concentrate on everyday processes such as appetite, digestion, urination, defecation and sleep. They take a dietary history and work to improve the diet and encourage other lifestyle changes. So they do make a diagnosis, but their system of doing so is different from that of Western medicine.

Are any herbal remedies recommended by conventional doctors?

Peppermint oil and aloe vera are frequently recommended and widely available without prescription for IBS.

What other herbal medicines are used for IBS?

Ginger is traditionally used for nausea. It is said to enhance emptying of the stomach while at the same time reducing spasm in the bowel. This should make it very useful for IBS, but surprisingly no studies have evaluated its efficacy. Iberogast (see below) is used for dyspepsia and IBS. Chinese herbal medicine is also widely available in the UK.

Does peppermint oil work in IBS?

The main active ingredient of peppermint oil is menthol. Applied to the smooth muscle of the intestine, menthol has a direct relaxing effect, reducing spasm. Peppermint oil is now so commonly used as an antispasmodic that it has acquired a place in conventional medicine. There are a number of small studies in people with IBS that mostly confirm a modest benefit over a placebo (dummy) treatment. There are usually no side effects, although a few people may complain of heartburn.

What is aloe vera, and does it work for IBS?

Aloe, or *Aloe vera*, is a cactus-like plant with a long history as a 'natural' remedy. Processing the leaves produces two compounds: aloe latex, or aloe juice, from the outer layer of the leaves, and aloe gel, which comes when the leaves are pulped. Aloe juice is a bitter-tasting, yellow fluid containing substances called anthraquinones. This makes it a stimulating laxative and it is used for this purpose (see Chapter 7 for a discussion on laxatives). Aloe gel is used as a non-greasy base for skin creams and is claimed to have therapeutic properties. The mechanical separation process is not always complete, so aloe latex can be found in some aloe gels.

Aloe gel has been claimed as a remedy for IBS, but there are no published studies on this. Nevertheless, I have seen people who have found it helpful as an antispasmodic, and it is often recommended as something to try, particularly in constipation-predominant IBS.

Does Chinese herbal medicine work?

Chinese herbal medicine is widely practised in the UK. Practitioners take a medical history and tailor the treatment to the individual's clinical presentation. Consequently, people with the same diagnosis may actually receive different treatments. This individualisation of treatment is common in complementary medicine and makes it difficult to scientifically test the effectiveness of particular treatments.

One interesting scientific study of Chinese herbal medicine for IBS in Australia was published in the *Journal of the American Medical Association* in 1998. In this study, 106 people with IBS were randomly divided into three treatment groups. One group received individualised Chinese herbal medicine, another received standard herbal Chinese medicine, and the third group received a placebo (inactive treatment). All the patients consulted a Chinese herbalist, and all the treatments were provided in capsules so that the people themselves and the gastroenterologists assessing them were unaware of who was receiving which treatment.

After 16 weeks of treatment, 33% of those receiving the placebo had improved, which is a typical result for an IBS study (for a discussion on the placebo effect, see earlier in the chapter). However, the Chinese herbs gave a significantly better result: 76% of those taking the standard Chinese herbs, and slightly less – 64% – of those with individualised herbal preparations improved with the treatment.

Moreover, the improvement seemed to last, and it lasted better in those who had received the individualised treatment. The study subjects were again assessed 14 weeks after the end of treatment. This time, 63% of the standard treatment group still felt improved, compared with 75% of the individualised treatment group and 32% of the placebo-treated group.

No serious side effects were noted during this study. Only two patients withdrew, one because of headaches and one because of gastrointestinal discomfort. Chinese medicine has been associated with liver function problems, but no such problem was noted here.

The authors concluded that Chinese herbal medicine worked for IBS, and that individualised treatment worked better. They suggested that the individualised Chinese herbal treatment may have been able to address the individuals' underlying problems, possibly by including herbs with sedative or anti-anxiety properties. The standard Chinese herbal medicine for IBS had no sedative properties and was a formulation considered to improve bowel function.

Surprisingly, I can find no other scientific studies of Chinese herbal medicine for IBS that have been published in English.

What is Iberogast, and might it work for my IBS?

Iberogast is a combination of herbs: bitter candytuft, chamomile flower, peppermint leaves, caraway fruit, licorice root, lemon balm leaves, celandine herbs, angelica root and milk thistle fruit.

A study from Germany published in 2003 compared the efficacy of Iberogast with a simplified six-herb preparation (bitter candytuft, chamomile flower, peppermint leaves, caraway fruit, licorice root and lemon balm leaves), with the single herb bitter candytuft and with a placebo (inactive treatment) in IBS. This was a reasonably large study with about 50 people randomly allocated to each group.

After 28 days of treatment, the result was judged to be good or very good in 38.5% of those receiving the placebo, which is typical of IBS studies. However, the Iberogast and the simplified six-herb preparation were significantly better – 64.7% of people in the study and 72.6% of physicians judged the efficacy to be good or very good. By contrast, the bitter candytuft on its own was no better than the placebo. There were no significant side effects from the herbal preparations, and the results of blood tests taken during the study remained normal.

Iberogast is available commercially in Europe and the USA. I sometimes suggest to people that they try it, although in the UK it is difficult to obtain and usually has to be ordered from abroad.

HYPNOSIS

What is hypnosis?

Hypnosis involves inducing a deeply relaxed state of mind in which the person's normal critical faculties are bypassed, allowing a state of heightened receptivity to suggestions. Once the person is in this state, sometimes called a hypnotic trance, the therapist makes therapeutic suggestions to encourage changes in behaviour or relieve symptoms.

Hypnosis is not sleep. Neither are subjects in a hypnotic state under the control of the hypnotist. The subject has to co-operate for the hypnotic state to be achieved. While the subject is hypnotised, he or she still has free will but has enhanced attention to what is being said. In conventional hypnosis, people approach the suggestions of the hypnotist, or their own ideas, as if they were reality. If the hypnotist suggests that your tongue has swollen up to twice its size, you'll feel a sensation like this in your mouth and you may have trouble talking.

How is this hypnotic state induced?

There are different methods of inducing hypnosis, but in every case subjects must want to be hypnotised. They must also believe that they can be hypnotised, and they must be made to feel comfortable and relaxed.

The fixed-gaze induction or eye-fixation method was popular in the early days of hypnosis and is the method we tend to see in films. The hypnotist waves a pocket watch in front of the subject. The idea is to get the subject to focus on an object so intently that he or she tunes out any other stimuli. As the subject focuses, the hypnotist talks to him or her in a low tone, lulling the subject into relaxation. However, this method does not work on a large proportion of the population.

The most common method used by therapists is called progressive relaxation and imagery. The hypnotist speaks to the subject in a slow, soothing voice, gradually bringing on complete relaxation and easing the subject into full hypnosis. Self-hypnosis training, as well as relaxation and meditation audiotapes, uses this method too.

What happens in gut-directed hypnotherapy?

Hypnosis as a treatment for IBS involves the use of what has been termed 'gut-directed hypnotherapy'. This was first developed by Dr P. J. Whorwell at the University Hospital of South Manchester in 1984 and currently comprises weekly 1-hour sessions for up to 12 weeks. Each session consists of inducing and deepening the hypnotic state, followed by 'ego-strengthening' suggestions relevant to the individual. These are accompanied by further suggestions and interventions, such as inducing warmth in the abdomen using the hands, and imagery directed towards controlling and normalising gut function. The sessions are supported by audiotapes used at home for self-hypnosis.

Does gut-directed hypnotherapy work for IBS?

Hypnotherapy cannot be evaluated in the same way as drug therapy. A double-blind placebo-controlled trial, which is what is used to evaluate conventional medicines (see above), is impossible because co-operation and rapport are needed between the client and therapist to achieve a hypnotic trance, and there is no such thing as a placebo hypnosis.

Even so, hypnosis for IBS has been studied extensively since 1984 and has proved to be superior to psychotherapy combined with placebo pills. Positive results for hypnotherapy have been consistently obtained in mostly non-randomised uncontrolled studies. In these studies, all the subjects get the same treatment, and the object is to see how many will benefit. The problem with such studies is that it is impossible to know whether the improvement is a real effect of the treatment or a placebo effect. (For an explanation of the placebo effect, see above.)

Even so, hypnotherapy seems to consistently improve the symptoms of IBS. Moreover, this improvement seems to be maintained. For example, in an audit of over 200 people with IBS treated with hypnotherapy in Manchester, 71% felt better at the end of the treatment. When they were reviewed by questionnaire 6 years later, 81% of those who had improved felt that this improvement had been maintained. To the best of my knowledge, no study has compared hypnosis with active medical treatment.

Can you give me some examples of the suggestions that are made to people while they are in a hypnotic state?

A person with constipation-predominant IBS might be asked to imagine the bowel as a river:

Imagine your bowel as a stagnant river, its water murky, polluted, foul-smelling, full of drifting rubbish that clogs its channels. Now see the river beginning to flow, gently at first, then faster and clearer, through green grassy meadows, with the sun shining overhead.

Similarly, for a person with diarrhoea:

Imagine your bowel as a river, flowing fast, raging through a canyon, swirling and bubbling. Now see the canyon opening into a valley, lush and green. The water slows, flowing serenely through quiet fields.

Is hypnosis safe?

Adverse reactions to hypnosis are rare. There are reports of hypnosis exacerbating psychological problems when unexpected thoughts and feelings come through during or after hypnosis. People may be distressed by reliving previous traumas, and there have been cases of 'false memories' being induced in psychologically vulnerable people. The most common suspected adverse reactions to hypnosis include drowsiness, dizziness, stiffness, headaches and anxiety.

How does hypnosis work?

We don't really know how hypnosis works. You can think of it as a form of psychological therapy that directly addresses the subconscious mind. That it works in IBS shows just how much the mind and body interact in this condition.

How available is hypnotherapy? Is it easy to get hypnotherapy?

Hypnotherapy is widely available in the UK but not usually on the NHS. It isn't difficult to find a hypnotherapist. You can search on Internet search engines such as Google for hypnosis, or gut-directed hypnotherapy, or look in the Yellow Pages. Some societies offer lists of therapists, their qualifications and the conditions they treat. These include the British Society of Clinical Hypnosis and the National Register of Hypnotherapists and Psychotherapists (see the Appendix for contact details). The problem is knowing whom to go to. There is a lack of effective regulation of hypnotherapists, and your family doctor or specialist may not know any of the local practitioners. It is best to contact the two societies above if you want to try this form of treatment.

ACUPUNCTURE

What is acupuncture?

Acupuncture has been used in China for over 2500 years. It began to achieve prominence in the West after an American journalist travelling with President Nixon to China in 1972 was treated successfully with acupuncture for complications after his appendix had been removed. Since then, it has gained considerable acceptance. Some family doctors and physiotherapists use acupuncture themselves, others refer patients, and many people refer themselves.

Acupuncture involves stimulating specific points on the skin by inserting needles. The needles are then used to stimulate these points mechanically or with a small electrical current. In traditional Chinese medicine, health is thought to depend on the body's 'motivating energy', called *Qi* (pronounced chee), moving in a smooth and balanced way through a series of channels beneath the skin; these channels are called meridians.

Qi consists of equal and opposite qualities – Yin and Yang – and when these become unbalanced, illness may result. By inserting fine needles into the channels of energy, an acupuncturist can alter the flow of Qi to restore its natural balance. The flow of Qi can be disturbed by a number of factors, including emotional states, poor nutrition, weather conditions, hereditary factors, infections, poisons and trauma. Acupuncture aims to restore the balance between the individual's physical, emotional and spiritual aspects.

Is there a difference between traditional Chinese acupuncture and the acupuncture used in the West?

Western-style or medical acupuncture, as practised mostly by doctors and physiotherapists, uses a more limited range of acupuncture techniques on the basis of a Western medical diagnosis. The Chinese concepts underlying acupuncture are largely not used. Instead, acupuncture points are thought to correspond to physiological and anatomical features or 'trigger points'; stimulating these leads to activation of parts of the central nervous system. There is some evidence for this from functional MRI (magnetic resonance imaging) and PET (positron electron tomography) brain scans. There is also some evidence that acupuncture causes the brain to release its own pain control molecules, called endorphins.

What is acupuncture used for?

A cupuncture appears to be effective for nausea and vomiting, especially after operations or chemotherapy. It is frequently used for chronic pain, although the evidence for its effectiveness is still inconclusive.

Is acupuncture used for IBS?

A cupuncture is used for IBS, but there is no evidence to say whether or not it is effective. There have been surprisingly few studies published in English, and only one double-blind study, the type of study that is best suited to seeing whether a treatment works (see earlier in the chapter for an explanation of a double-blind study). In that study, 25 patients at a hospital in Israel each had four acupuncture treatments – two true treatments and two sham treatments with needles placed at the 'wrong' acupuncture points. The first true treatment led to a significant improvement in symptoms compared with the first sham treatment. However, the second true treatment was ineffective, so the study was inconclusive.

Are there any side effects with acupuncture?

S erious side effects such as viral hepatitis B infection caught from a needle, or a collapsed lung after it has been penetrated by a needle, have been reported but are very rare. In one study of Swedish physiotherapists, minor bleeding or bruising occurred after nearly one in five treatments. Headache, fainting, nausea or fatigue have been reported to occur after about one in a thousand treatments.

COLONIC HYDROTHERAPY

What is colonic hydrotherapy?

Colonic hydrotherapy, or colonic irrigation, involves water at a very low pressure and a controlled temperature being slowly introduced into the colon through a tube passed into the rectum through the anus (the back passage). It is performed by a trained therapist, often in combination with abdominal massage. The idea is to wash away faecal matter and pipe it away with the waste water. There is no mess and no smell. A colonic treatment lasts between 45 and 60 minutes.

Are there any side effects?

During colonic irrigation, the colon muscles will sometimes contract suddenly, expelling considerable amounts of liquid and waste into the rectum. This may feel like cramping or gas, and may create a feeling of urgency to empty the rectum. Such episodes, if they do occur, are brief and easily tolerated. There are no reports of any serious side effects.

Does colonic hydrotherapy work for IBS?

There are no studies on this, so it is difficult to comment. I have had several patients with difficult constipation who have benefitted. I imagine that, for most people, laxatives would have a similar effect. The laxatives that we use to prepare the bowel before a barium enema or colonoscopy usually leave it sparkling clean!

CONCLUSION

As a hard-and-fast scientist, I often tend to be sceptical about the underlying theories and assumptions of complementary medicine. A large part of the benefit that some people experience may be attributable to the placebo effect – their belief in their therapist and the treatment – rather than being a true effect of the treatment. I sometimes see people who use a different complementary medicine every few months, enthuse about each until the benefit wears off and then move on to another therapy. But does it really matter if they are benefitting from a placebo effect as long as they feel better? Doesn't this just show what positive thinking can do?

Medicine clearly has much to discover, and it is likely that some complementary medicines will find a place within conventional medicine. How they work will be determined, the active ingredients will be purified, and the side effects and risks will undoubtedly be documented.

People tend to believe that complementary medicines are harmless, whereas conventional drugs have side effects. But we know about the side effects of these drugs as they have been extensively tested and regulated. This is not, however, the case with complementary medicine. We simply don't know what effects they may have in the short or long term. A potent treatment without the risk of side effects is unfortunately as rare as a free lunch! Even so, it is unusual to see a patient who has been harmed by complementary medicine.

As we've seen many times in this book, treating IBS is often a matter of experimenting, and I generally encourage people to try treatments that appeal to them, as we can't predict what will work in each individual case.

SUMMARY

- Most complementary treatments have not been tested to anything like the same degree as conventional treatments.

- Their proponents feel that the scientific model used in medicine may not apply to complementary treatments.

- Complementary treatments are mostly used in conditions that are not well served by conventional medicines.

- We all see people who have benefited from complementary medicine.

- The benefit of complementary treatments may lie to a large extent in the placebo effect – we don't yet know.

- Some complementary treatments have been tested in IBS patients with positive results, but such studies have been few in number and of a small scale.

- The complementary treatments that have some evidence of efficacy in IBS include gut-directed hypnotherapy, Chinese medicine, peppermint oil and Iberogast.

- We are unlikely for some time to have information on how well these treatments work. In the meantime, the placebo effect alone shows the enormous power of positive thinking, and you may also derive extra benefits.

13 | Medical tests and investigations: what they involve and what they mean

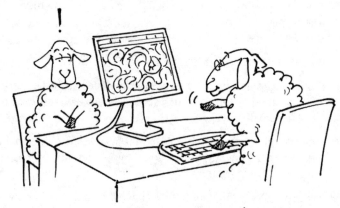

'Hmm... your bowel conditions are actually closer to El Nino than IBS...'

In previous centuries, the doctor was a wise old soul who looked at the patient and pontificated from the end of the bed. In the words of Benjamin Franklin, 'God heals, and the doctor takes the fee'! Today, modern medicine is dominated by tests, sometimes snobbishly called investigations. To some people, the thought of these tests is worse than the disease. To others, normal test results are so reassuring that they are actually therapeutic.

Table 13.1 Some factors that influence the extent
of medical investigation for IBS

Factor	Comment
Length of time that the symptoms have been present	The longer the symptoms have been present without progressing, the less likely it is that serious disease is present
Age	Cancer is unusual under the age of 50. Very old or frail people will tolerate the tests less well
Family history	The average lifetime risk of bowel cancer is about 1 in 25. However, having just one first-degree relative (a parent or sibling) with bowel cancer doubles that risk. If you have a first-degree relative with inflammatory bowel disease (Crohn's disease or ulcerative colitis), this increases your risk of getting inflammatory bowel disease to about 1 in 10
Weight loss	This is unusual in IBS
Bleeding from the back passage	This does not happen in IBS
Diarrhoea at night	This is unusual in IBS
Diarrhoea that fails to respond to loperamide (see Chapter 8)	This is unusual in IBS
Constipation	Constipation is much less likely than diarrhoea to represent serious pathology
Your doctor's attitude	Some doctors investigate more than others
Your own attitude	Some people are more tolerant of uncertainty than others. And some people are less tolerant of medical tests than others

I understand that there are no specific tests for IBS, so why do I need any test at all?

You don't necessarily 'need' any test at all. Medical investigations (tests) for irritable bowel syndrome (IBS) are all about reducing the chance of a mistaken diagnosis, reducing uncertainty. The degree of uncertainty depends on a number of factors, including how long the symptoms have been present, how typical they are of IBS, your age and your family history (Table 13.1). As there can never be absolute certainty, the extent of your medical investigation will ultimately depend on how much uncertainty you and your doctor are happy with.

What tests might be used to investigate abdominal symptoms?

In this chapter, I will briefly describe some of the large variety of tests available: what they involve, what they show, how doctors choose between different investigations and the limitations of these tests. Some of the investigations used in gastroenterology (gut medicine) are given in Table 13.2. Figure 1.1 in Chapter 1 shows where most of the different parts of the gut can be found.

COLONOSCOPY

What is a colonoscopy?

The term 'colonoscopy' means looking inside the colon. The colon, or large bowel, is the last portion of your digestive (gastro-intestinal) tract (Figure 13.1). It starts in the lower right corner of the abdomen, where it is attached to the end of the small intestine. This part of the colon is called the caecum. It ends at the rectum and anus. The colon is a hollow tube, about 1–2 metres long, whose main function is to store unabsorbed food products before their elimination.

Table 13.2 Investigations used in gastroenterology

	Comment
Endoscopic procedures	
Gastroscopy	Examines the oesophagus, stomach and duodenum
Colonoscopy	Examines the large bowel (colon), from the anus to the caecum
Flexible sigmoidoscopy	Examines just the lower 40 centimetres of the bowel from the anus upwards
ERCP (endoscopic retrograde cholangiopancreatography)	Examines the bile duct and the pancreatic duct
Endoscopic capsule	A new technique to look at the small bowel
Radiological procedures	
Plain abdominal X-ray	Can demonstrate small or large bowel obstruction. Can also show severe constipation
Barium enema	Examines the large bowel (colon)
Barium follow-through	Examines the small bowel
Virtual colonoscopy	Examines the large bowel (colon). Uses a sophisticated CT (computed tomography) scanner and complicated software to create a computer-generated three-dimensional picture of the colon. It has recently been invented and is not yet widely available
Ultrasound scan of the abdomen	Examines the liver, gall bladder, bile ducts, kidneys, aorta (the main artery to the body) and pancreas
CT scan of the abdomen	Similar to ultrasound but more detailed

Table 13.2 Investigations used in gastroenterology *continued*

	Comment
Blood tests	
Full blood count (FBC)	One of the most important tests. It will demonstrate anaemia (too few red blood cells) and may suggest a cause such as iron deficiency
ESR (erythrocyte sedimentation rate) and CRP (C-reactive protein level)	A high ESR or CRP means that there is too much inflammation somewhere in the body. Results are normal in IBS but often abnormal in inflammatory bowel disease (Crohn's disease or ulcerative colitis)
Urea, creatinine and electrolytes (commonly referred to as Us & Es)	Denote renal function. They may indicate dehydration
Glucose	In its early stages, the symptoms of diabetes can be subtle and the only clue will be a higher level of glucose in the blood
Amylase	Blood amylase levels are very high in acute pancreatitis (severe inflammation of the pancreas)
Liver function tests (LFTs)	Ongoing serious liver disease may have no symptoms but can be detected with these tests. Unfortunately, they often show minor abnormalities that cause great concern but turn out to be irrelevant
Thyroid function tests (TFTs)	Thyroid function abnormalities are fairly common. Symptoms can be subtle and frequently affect gut function
Coeliac screen	Coeliac disease may affect as many as 1 in 100 people, causing a wide variety of symptoms often mistaken for IBS. A negative blood test makes coeliac disease very unlikely

Table 13.2 Investigations used in gastroenterology *continued*

	Comment
Stool tests	
Microscopy and culture	Will usually detect some infective causes of diarrhoea such as *Campylobacter* and *Salmonella*, and will occasionally detect *Giardia*. It will not detect viral infections or small bowel bacterial overgrowth (see Chapter 8)
Clostridium difficile toxin	Used to detect a severe type of antibiotic-related diarrhoea called pseudomembranous colitis
Faecal occult blood	A very sensitive test that will detect tiny amounts of blood in the stool. It may be used as a screening test for bowel cancer. Unfortunately, it is often positive in the absence of significant disease (called a false-positive result)
Faecal microscopy for fat	Excess fat seen in the stool denotes a problem with the digestion or absorption of fat. This occurs in coeliac disease and pancreatic disease

The instrument that is used to look inside the colon is the colonoscope (Figure 13.1). This is a long, thin, flexible tube with a tiny video camera and a light on the end. By adjusting the various controls on the colonoscope, the doctor or nurse can carefully guide the instrument in any direction to look at the inside of the colon. A high-quality picture from the colonoscope is shown on a TV monitor. Other instruments can be passed through the colonoscope, so samples of tissue (biopsies) can be taken to examine under a microscope (histology). You won't usually feel anything while the tissue is being removed.

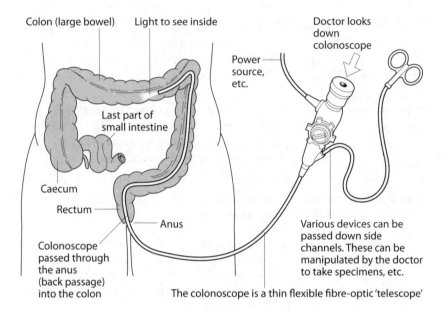

Figure 13.1 Colonoscopy.

What sort of abnormalities can a colonoscopy detect?

Colonoscopy is the best technique currently available to detect any abnormality in the colon. It is predominantly used to look for problems such as cancer, inflammation (red, swollen patches) or polyps. Polyps are small lumps, like cherries, on the inside wall of the bowel. Diverticular disease is easily seen as small pouches arising from the bowel wall. Small abnormal blood vessels (angiodysplasia) within the wall of bowel can be seen if the bowel is clean.

Preparing for a colonoscopy

Your bowel has to be cleared out before a colonoscopy. You do this at home, usually the day before. Your endoscopy unit will give you the necessary laxatives (medicines to empty the bowel, but considerably more potent than those you buy at the chemist) and a list of instructions. These vary somewhat between different units, but it is important that you read and follow these instructions.

For many patients, clearing the bowel can be the most trying part of the entire test. It is vital though that you complete this step carefully, because how well the bowel is emptied determines how successful the procedure is. If your bowel isn't clean, it will be difficult or impossible for the doctor or nurse to guide the colonoscope around your colon. The procedure will also take longer to perform, and there will be a greater risk of a problem being missed. In some cases, you might have to have a repeat procedure.

Clearing out the bowel usually involves:

- no solid food for 24 hours;

- powerful laxatives taken over 24 hours;

- drinking a large volume of water (about 3–5 litres, or 5–9 pints);

- passing large amounts of loose stool.

What can I expect during my colonoscopy?

Before the procedure, you will obviously need to take off most of your clothes and change into a hospital gown. An intravenous, or IV, line will be inserted to give you medication to make you feel relaxed and drowsy. This is *not* a general anaesthetic. The drug will enable you to stay awake and co-operative, but you will usually be too drowsy to remember much of the experience. Your pulse and the oxygen content of your blood will be continuously monitored using a sensor placed on a finger. You will lie on your left side with your knees pulled into your chest.

Once you are fully relaxed, your doctor will do a rectal examination with a gloved, lubricated finger, and the lubricated colonoscope will then be gently inserted. As this is slowly and carefully passed in, you may feel as if you need to move your bowels, and because air is introduced to help advance the colonoscope, you may feel some cramping or fullness. The extent of the discomfort varies greatly between people, but there is generally little or no discomfort.

The colonoscope and the air introduced through it inevitably stretch and distend the bowel. Some people, especially those with IBS, are more sensitive to distension of the bowel and may suffer more discomfort. As the colonoscope is withdrawn from the bowel, as much air as possible is sucked out through the instrument, leaving you as comfortable as possible. The time needed for colonoscopy varies, but on the average the procedure takes about 30 minutes.

Does it matter who performs the colonoscopy?

Colonoscopy is a highly skilled procedure, more so than many other procedures. Although there is now much more emphasis on formal training than there was previously, there are still significant variations in skill between practitioners. This may mean that the colonoscopy takes a longer time to complete or that there is more discomfort. Most importantly, however, it is reflected in the completion rate – the percentage of times that the operator manages to get the colonoscope all the way around the colon to see the caecum. Completion rates ought to be above 90%, but surveys in the UK have suggested that they may fall as low as 70%.

What happens if the colonoscopy is not completed?

Even in the best hands, it may not be possible to get the colonoscope all the way round to the caecum, for a number of reasons: the bowel may be very long, with many twists and turns; there may be severe diverticular disease (see Chapter 5), which makes colonoscopy both more difficult and more risky; the bowel may not be sufficiently clean; or the procedure may be causing the patient too much discomfort and the doctor may feel that more sedation is too risky.

A further procedure may be necessary to complete looking at the bowel. This may mean another colonoscopy or a barium enema.

What are the possible complications from a colonoscopy?

Although colonoscopy is a safe procedure, complications can sometimes occur. These include perforation – a puncture of the wall of the colon – which might require surgical repair. The average risk of a perforation is about 1 in 1000, but this increases if there is severe diverticular disease, or if polyps (small lumps on the inside of your colon) need to be removed. When a polyp removal (polypectomy) or biopsy is performed, there is sometimes heavy bleeding (haemorrhage), which may need a blood transfusion or reinsertion of the colonoscope to control the bleeding. The risk of a significant bleed after a polypectomy is about 1 in 200.

The sedatives and painkillers given to make the procedure more tolerable can affect a person's breathing and heart, but serious problems are rare because breathing is monitored during the colonoscopy. Blood pressure may be monitored too.

What can I expect after my colonoscopy?

Afterwards, you'll be cared for in a recovery area until the effects of the medication have mostly worn off. At this time, you will be informed about the results of your colonoscopy and provided with any additional information that you need. It is normally possible to eat and drink as soon as the sedation has worn off.

Occasionally, minor problems may persist, such as bloating, gas or mild cramping. But these symptoms should disappear in 24 hours or less. By the time you are ready to go home, you will feel stronger and more alert. Nevertheless, you should rest for the remainder of the day.

You need to have a family member or friend take you home. If there is no one to help you home, you will not be given sedation.

Tips for a successful colonoscopy

Take all your laxatives. If you lose them, vomit them or inadvertently pour them down the sink, contact your endoscopy unit. They may be able to get you more laxatives in time, but if not, it may be better to postpone the procedure.

Drink plenty of fluids while taking the laxatives. This will keep you hydrated and help cleanse your bowel.

Use an ointment to protect your anus while taking the laxatives, otherwise you will become sore. Any haemorrhoid preparation or nappy rash cream will do. Petroleum jelly (Vaseline) is the simplest choice.

Don't be embarrassed. The doctor and his team will concentrate so much on the inside of your colon that they will not really notice any other part of your anatomy. And try not to worry. In general, fewer than 10% of patients are found to have a cancer at colonoscopy.

Don't be surprised if you can't remember much of what happened. One of the drugs most commonly used for sedation (Midazolam) has an amnesic effect – an effect that makes you forget.

And don't plan to do anything special the following day. You may feel great, but you may also feel a little tired, and may still have windy pains from air left in your bowel.

FLEXIBLE SIGMOIDOSCOPY

A flexible sigmoidoscopy is like a colonoscopy but uses a shorter tube. So it's useful only for looking inside your rectum and the lowest part of your colon (called the sigmoid colon). This test finds up to two-thirds of polyps (small lumps on the inside of your bowel) and cancers. You may have a sigmoidoscopy if you have:

- bright red bleeding from your anus, not the darker bleeding that looks like it comes from higher up in your bowel;
- pain in the left side of your abdomen.

You don't need to clean out your whole bowel with laxatives before a sigmoidoscopy. Instead, you get an enema that cleans out just the lower part of the bowel.

Flexible sigmoidoscopy usually does not require sedation. If you feel that you would like sedation, make a point of asking for it.

BARIUM ENEMA

This is a method of visualising the bowel with X-rays. The gut does not show up very well on ordinary X-ray pictures. However, if it is coated with barium, it shows up clearly outlined by white. This is because X-rays do not pass through barium but are instead absorbed by it. Barium is a soft, white metal, and a compound of barium called barium sulphate dissolves in water to form a thick white liquid. Unfortunately, you still have to clear out your bowel beforehand in the same way as for a colonoscopy.

The procedure is performed in the X-ray department. A thick, white liquid that contains the barium sulphate is passed up a tube into your back passage, and air is pumped in to distend the bowel. The barium sticks to the lining of your bowel. When the barium absorbs the X-rays and pictures are taken, they show an outline of the inside of the bowel. In this way, cancers, polyps, diverticular disease and other conditions are shown up. A series of pictures will be taken as the barium liquid passes back down your bowel. You will be moved into various positions to facilitate different views. Distending the bowel with air may be a little uncomfortable, but no sedation is necessary.

Your stools may be white for a few days after a barium enema. This is the barium liquid leaving your body, and it's nothing to worry about. This test is very safe, but some people get spasmy pains in their abdomen, and there is a very small risk that part of the wall of your bowel could puncture, causing a perforation. This risk is very small indeed, much smaller than the 1 in 1000 risk of perforation quoted for colonoscopy.

What are the differences between a colonoscopy and a barium enema?

Table 13.3 describes these differences.

Table 13.3 Differences between a colonoscopy and a barium enema

	Colonoscopy	Barium enema
Preparation	No difference	No difference
Sedation	Conscious sedation	No sedation
Discomfort	Usually minimal with sedation	Minimal
Accuracy	It is more accurate, and allows lesions to be biopsied (samples taken) and polyps to be removed	It is less accurate, especially in the rectum and sigmoid colon. It can miss small lesions
Completion	In good hands, the caecum wil be visualised in over 90% of people	It will almost always visualise the caecum
Will further procedures be necessary?	A barium enema may be necessary if the colonoscopy is incomplete	Flexible sigmoidoscopy is often performed to see the rectum and sigmoid colon better. If a suspicious lesion, a cancer or a polyp is seen, a colonoscopy will be performed to remove the polyp or to take biopsies
Risk of bowel perforation	Low, about 1 in 1000	Very low. It is safer than a colonoscopy
Side effects after the test	Drowsiness from the sedation Abdominal cramping from the residual air	More cramping from the residual air (at colonoscopy most of the air is sucked out as the instrument is withdrawn). Barium can be constipating

There seem to be quite a few tests that can be done. How do doctors decide whether to do a colonoscopy, a barium enema, a flexible sigmoidoscopy or both a flexible sigmoidoscopy and a barium enema?

This decision depends mainly on the person's symptoms and partly on whether the test is easily available at the local hospital.

If the symptoms are limited to the left side of the bowel, for example only left-sided pain or bright red rectal bleeding, a flexible sigmoidoscopy will allow all the relevant areas to be seen.

If the problem is mainly pain occurring on both sides of the abdomen, the main function of the test is to rule out a cancer causing a blockage in the bowel. A barium enema on its own is usually entirely satisfactory.

If the problem is mainly diarrhoea, with or without pain, it could be inflammatory bowel disease (Crohn's disease or ulcerative colitis), and this can be seen better with a colonoscopy.

If the problem is anaemia, we usually prefer a colonoscopy. Any polyps (small lumps on the inside of your bowel wall) that may have been bleeding can be removed, biopsies (samples) can be taken from tumours, and small abnormal blood vessels that may have been bleeding can sometimes be seen too.

If the waiting list for colonoscopy is too long, or if your colon is known to be difficult to get through, the doctor may choose a combination of flexible sigmoidoscopy and a barium enema. The flexible sigmoidoscopy is good at seeing the rectum and sigmoid colon, where up to two-thirds of polyps and cancers can be found. The barium enema is good at looking at the rest of the bowel.

GASTROSCOPY

This is also called an upper GI (gastrointestinal) endoscopy, or just an endoscopy.

What's the difference between an endoscopy and a gastroscopy?

'Endoscopy' is the general term for an examination of an interior canal or a hollow organ using a special instrument. Gastroscopy – examination of the stomach – was the first endoscopy to be routinely performed, and the two terms are often used synonymously.

What is a gastroscopy?

The term 'gastroscopy' just means looking inside the stomach. In fact, the procedure actually involves looking at the entire upper gastrointestinal tract, including the oesophagus, the stomach and the duodenum (Figure 13.2).

An endoscope called a gastroscope is used. It is similar in design to a colonoscope but is usually slimmer and more flexible. There are a video camera and light at the end of the endoscope, and a high-quality image is generated on a TV monitor. As with most endoscopes, there is an extra channel for passing instruments so that treatments can be carried out and biopsies (samples) taken.

What's a gastroscopy used for?

A gastroscopy is used to check for and treat ulcers, cancers or bleeding blood vessels in the upper gastrointestinal tract. It is also used for taking biopsies of the small bowel to diagnose coeliac disease (sensitivity to gluten).

How do I prepare for a gastroscopy?

Gastroscopies take place in the hospital's endoscopy unit. You will be asked not to eat anything for at least 4 hours before your gastroscopy because food can stop the doctor from seeing inside your stomach. You will be able to have a few sips of water for up to 2 hours before your test. If you do eat something, your test may need to be cancelled or delayed.

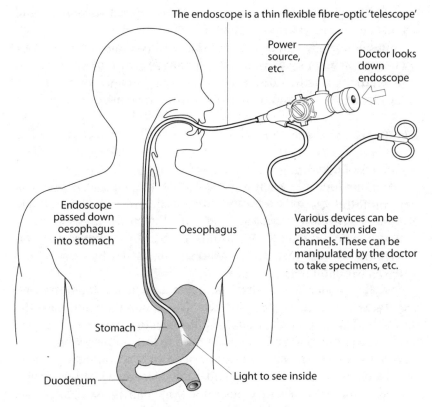

The endoscope is a thin flexible fibre-optic 'telescope'

Power source, etc.

Doctor looks down endoscope

Endoscope passed down oesophagus into stomach

Oesophagus

Various devices can be passed down side channels. These can be manipulated by the doctor to take specimens, etc.

Stomach

Duodenum

Light to see inside

Figure 13.2 Gastroscopy.

What happens during the test?

Most units offer people a choice of sedation or no sedation. If you choose not to have sedation, you will get a spray for the back of your mouth that will somewhat numb the back of your mouth and throat, and reduce your gag reflex. If you choose to have sedation, an intravenous, or IV, line will be inserted to give you the medication to make you relaxed and drowsy. This is *not* a general anaesthetic. The drug will enable you to remain awake and co-operative, but you will usually be too drowsy to remember much of the experience.

You will need to lie on your left side during the procedure. Your doctor or nurse will give you a plastic mouth guard to put between your teeth. This is to stop your teeth being damaged by the endoscope and to stop you biting it. You will need to breathe through your nose during the test, although it is usually still possible to mouth-breathe if your nose is blocked. Your pulse and the oxygen content of your blood will be continuously monitored using a sensor placed on one of your fingers.

The endoscope will be guided over the back of your tongue. It will feel as though you have a lump at the back of your throat. You will be asked to 'swallow' as this action opens the top of the oesophagus. Even if you do not manage to swallow properly, the endoscopist can normally guide the instrument behind your larynx (voice box) and into your oesophagus.

To make it easier to see what's going on, air will be blown through the endoscope as it is passed down the oesophagus and into the stomach. This can make you feel bloated, and you may want to belch. This is normal, and you don't need to feel embarrassed.

In some cases, it may be necessary to take a sample of tissue, called a biopsy, to examine later under the microscope. This is a painless procedure. If necessary, the endoscope can be used to treat a problem such as active bleeding from an ulcer.

A gastroscopy usually takes about 10 minutes.

Should I have my gastroscopy with or without sedation?

It's a personal choice. Without sedation, you will be aware of all that is going on and be in a better position to understand and discuss the results. You will be able to leave the endoscopy unit sooner and continue with your normal day. In general, about one third of people who have a gastroscopy without sedation say that it caused them minimal discomfort. Unfortunately, another third feel a lot of discomfort. It is impossible to predict how it will be for you until the procedure is underway, by which time it is too late to change your mind.

What can I expect after the gastroscopy?

You should not have any pain after a gastroscopy, although you may have a sore throat that occasionally lasts a day or two. You may feel a bit bloated and uncomfortable for a short time because of the air put into your stomach. If you have not had a sedative, you may only need 15–30 minutes to recover, and then you can go home or back to work. But you will not be able to eat or drink until the local anaesthetic spray has worn off (about an hour).

If you have had a sedative, it may take you about an hour before you stop feeling drowsy. You may not remember very much about the test afterwards. Sedatives can slow your reactions down so you will not be able to drive, and you will need someone to help you get home.

Your doctor or nurse may tell you what was found during the gastroscopy before you go home. For example, you may have an ulcer or inflammation in the oesophagus from acid reflux. But if samples of tissue (biopsies) were taken, you will have to wait for the results. Sometimes the hospital sends your results to your GP, but some people have to come back to an outpatient clinic for their results.

What are the risks of gastroscopy?

The risks of a routine gastroscopy are low; complications rarely occur. If they do, they include perforation – a puncture of the wall of the oesophagus, stomach or duodenum – which could require surgical repair, and bleeding, which could require a transfusion. The risk of a serious adverse event is probably about 1 in 1000.

What are the alternatives to gastroscopy?

A barium meal test is sometimes used instead of gastroscopy. During a barium meal, you are given a white liquid to drink.

This contains a metal called barium in a solution as barium sulphate. Barium sticks to the lining of your throat, stomach and intestine, and absorbs X-rays. This means that these parts of your body show up as white on an X-ray film. Doctors can then look at the X-ray film to see if there is anything unusual.

A barium meal is safer and easier than a gastroscopy but it is not as good at finding out what's wrong. This is because doctors cannot take a sample of tissue (biopsy) like they can during a gastroscopy. A barium meal picks up just over half of all ulcers, whereas gastroscopy picks up more than 9 in 10. So if you have a barium meal and the doctor thinks that there may be something wrong, you may have to have a gastroscopy afterwards.

BARIUM FOLLOW-THROUGH

This test is similar to a barium meal but aims to look for problems in the small intestine such as Crohn's disease. So you drink the barium solution but then you need to wait 10–15 minutes before any X-rays are taken. This allows time for the barium to reach the small intestine. You may then have an X-ray every 30 minutes or so until the barium is seen to have gone through all the small intestine and reached the large intestine (colon).

ULTRASOUND SCANS

What are ultrasound scans?

Ultrasound scans are images of the internal organs created from sound waves. The high-frequency sound waves are emitted by a hand-held transducer that is held on the skin and directed towards the organ being studied. Reflections of these sound waves are detected in the same transducer and converted into black and white images on a TV screen. Hard tissues such as bone reflect the biggest echoes and are white in the image; soft tissues appear grey and speckled. Fluids do not reflect any echoes so appear black. It is important to come to the scan with an empty stomach, otherwise food and air in the stomach will reduce the quality of the image.

What can an abdominal ultrasound show?

An abdominal ultrasound may be used to detect a large number of abnormalities, including gall stones, obstruction of the bile ducts by gall stones or tumours, kidney abnormalities such as tumours or obstruction of the kidney, liver abnormalities such as tumours, and large blood vessel abnormalities such as an abnormal enlargement of the aorta (aneurysm). Sometimes a good view of the pancreas is seen, but at other times the pancreas may be obscured by gas in bowel lying on top of it.

Ultrasound cannot give good views of the stomach, the small bowel or the large bowel.

CT (COMPUTED TOMOGRAPHY) SCANS

An abdominal CT scan gives more detailed views of the organs in the abdomen than an ultrasound scan does. However, it takes more time, uses more expensive machinery and involves a small dose of radiation. It does not give such good views of the stomach and bowel as endoscopy, but it does show the outside of the bowel and stomach. So, for example, it can tell whether a tumour found in the stomach has spread to adjacent organs.

ENDOSCOPIC CAPSULES

Invented in Israel, the endoscopic capsule measures 11 millimetres by 26 millimetres and weighs less than 4 g. It contains a light source, a camera, a transmitter and a battery. After being swallowed whole, it takes two pictures a second for 5–6 hours and transmits them to a receiver worn on a belt. The pictures are collected by a computer to make a 1–2 hour video. Eventually, the capsule passes harmlessly with the stool. It is not reused.

Because the capsule cannot be manoeuvred, it cannot provide such a good view of large, hollow organs such as the stomach or the large bowel. It is therefore not a substitute for gastroscopy or colonoscopy. The small bowel, however, is narrow enough for the capsule to provide a full view all the way round as it passes through. In this respect, it has proved to be markedly better than a barium follow-through. It is mainly used in people who are strongly suspected to have Crohn's disease but in whom all investigations, including barium follow-through and colonoscopy, have been normal.

PROBLEMS AND SOLUTIONS

I have had IBS symptoms for many years. My new family doctor referred me to a hospital specialist who has ordered a colonoscopy. There hasn't been a significant change in my symptoms over the years. Is there really any point in having this test now?

There are two ways of looking at this. You could argue that as nothing very much different has happened over the years – no significant weight loss, no bleeding etc. – the chance of the colonoscopy finding a cancer or inflammatory bowel disease (Crohn's disease or ulcerative colitis) is very low. And this is indeed true.

Moreover, you may suspect that the doctor has ordered the test for the wrong reason. Because you were referred, he may wrongly have assumed that you had got significantly worse. Perhaps he thought you were plagued by anxiety about cancer. Perhaps you feel that he has ordered the colonoscopy because that is what he always does with IBS patients. You may even uncharitably suspect that the doctor was just fobbing you off with a test because he couldn't think of anything else to do! These are all good reasons not to have a colonoscopy.

On the other hand, you could argue that IBS has been with you for a long time, so it is likely to stay. What concerns you is that, with increasing age, other conditions may have developed. It is possible that you have come to interpret the symptoms of the new condition as IBS. In other words, the IBS may be 'masking' another condition. There may also be some new stresses in your life that are making it more difficult to tolerate any uncertainty over your health. These are all good reasons to go ahead with the colonoscopy. Ultimately, it is your choice.

I have very bad veins. They always have trouble taking my blood.

Dress warmly, especially on your upper body. When you are hot, the blood supply to the skin increases, and the veins become more prominent. If you have a 'good' vein, be sure to recommend it.

I have a very sore anus. I'm afraid it will really hurt when examined.

Tell this to the doctor or nurse and they will use a jelly containing local anaesthetic.

I've taken all the laxatives that were sent to me in preparation for a colonoscopy, but they have not worked well. I'm still passing stool, or at best dirty looking water.

Tell this to the nurses when you arrive at the endoscopy unit. They will probably give you an enema to help clean your bowel.

I've been getting a lot of spasmy pains and bloating after my colonoscopy [or barium enema]. What can I do?

It's probably air in your bowel. It will pass. An antispasmodic such as peppermint oil may help.

I don't have anyone to take me home or stay with me after the colonoscopy. What should I do?

Tell the endoscopy unit. You can have the colonoscopy performed without sedation using gas and air (entenox), sometimes called laughing gas, to reduce the discomfort.

I was once sexually abused. I'm terrified of anyone approaching my anus.

Tell your doctor or nurse. There are simple things that they can do to make it easier. They can give you a sleeping tablet for the night before, or a small dose of valium or other sedative to take before leaving your home. They can also put you first on the list so that you don't have to wait too long. And they may be able to arrange for a woman to perform your test.

I'm afraid of having a gastroscopy. I have a very strong gag reflex. I don't think I will be able to swallow the tube.

This is a common concern that rarely turns out to be a problem. We can nearly always guide the endoscope into the oesophagus. If you are very nervous, we can sometimes give you more sedation.

Do people with IBS suffer more distress during and after procedures such as gastroscopy, flexible sigmoidoscopy or colonoscopy?

This is something that many gastroenterologists and patients believe may be true, although it has not been formally tested. In IBS the gut may be more sensitive to being distended. Any procedure that looks within the gut will involve distending it with air and to some extent stretching it as the instrument is passed, and some suffering is probably inevitable. Any air left behind following the procedure will also be less well tolerated in people with IBS.

However, with this suffering comes a better understanding of the condition. To some people, it is useful and reassuring to watch their normal bowel on the monitor during the procedure and note that their discomfort increases when the bowel is inflated with air, or when the instrument passes around a bend in the bowel (this usually causes some stretching).

Can I state a preference for how much sedation I get?

Most doctors and nurses will be happy to let you choose between mild, heavy or no sedation, as long as it's appropriate to the procedure being performed.

I'm a regular alcohol drinker (not excessive). Is it true that the sedation used for endoscopic procedures may be less effective for me and that consequently I may be more awake than I would like to be?

This is true. Regular alcohol consumption may make you more resistant to the effects of the commonly used sedatives. Higher doses will often work, but doctors and nurses are reluctant to use large doses, partly for fear of side effects, and partly for fear of breaking the now ubiquitous guidelines and protocols.

Why can't I have a general anaesthetic for the procedure?

General anaesthetics carry a small but significant risk because they render you unconscious with your reflexes suppressed. Conscious sedation that leaves you conscious but drowsy, and with your reflexes intact, is safer in most circumstances. There is also an economic argument as the timing and resources needed for a general anaesthetic would make the procedure much more expensive. General anaesthetics are usually only used for endoscopy in children.

CONCLUSION

Modern medicine puts a greater emphasis on diagnosing conditions early than ever before. In gastroenterology, the number of endoscopies (gastroscopies, flexible sigmoidoscopies and colonoscopies) we perform increases every year. We are predominantly looking for cancers in their early stages, when they can be more easily treated and cured. We inevitably subject people to fairly intrusive and unpleasant tests even though their symptoms may actually be quite mild. Some people have these tests even though they are completely well as part of screening. It is no surprise therefore that most of the results of these tests turn out to be normal. Even when family doctors send their patients for urgent endoscopies because they suspect a cancer, a cancer is found in only about 1 in 10 of such patients.

Part of the unpleasantness of these tests is the fear of what might be found. But most of these tests are normal or show minor abnormalities. The chance of a serious abnormality, such as a cancer, being found is usually less than 1 in 10. It is important to remember this fact because it is easy for people to assume that their doctor would never have ordered such tests unless there was a much greater probability of a serious problem. This may have been true in the past, but today most tests are performed for the reassurance that you are not the one with the cancer.

SUMMARY

- There is no specific test for IBS.
- People with IBS have medical tests to exclude other conditions.
- The most common organ to be looked at in people with IBS is the colon.

- The most common reason to look at the colon in people with IBS is to exclude inflammatory bowel disease (Crohn's disease or ulcerative colitis) or a cancer.

- The most common finding with a colonoscopy or flexible sigmoidoscopy is a normal bowel.

- The most common abnormal finding with a colonoscopy or flexible sigmoidoscopy is diverticular disease (see Chapter 5).

- The most common finding with a gastroscopy is a normal stomach.

- The most common abnormal finding with a gastroscopy is gastritis (inflammation in the stomach from excess acid or infection with *Helicobacter pylori*; see Chapter 5).

- The small bowel can be examined using a barium follow-through or an endoscopic capsule.

- The small bowel is examined much less frequently than the large bowel because cancer in the small bowel is rare.

- Some discomfort is inevitable with any test, but the nursing and medical staff are experienced in minimising your discomfort and embarrassment.

- Sedation is frequently used, but is not always necessary for endoscopic tests.

- Sedation is not a general anaesthetic. You remain awake but are usually too drowsy to remember much.

- Some people would prefer to put up with some uncertainty about their condition rather than undergo endoscopic tests. This is something to discuss with your doctor before coming for the test.

- The most important thing you can do for a successful test is to follow the instructions that you have been given as closely as possible.

- The most important thing to remember is that most of these tests find nothing seriously wrong.

Glossary

acute This usually means of rapid onset and brief. Occasionally, it is loosely used to mean severe.

aerophagia Air swallowing. The major source of stomach gas.

aetiology The scientific study of the causes of a disease.

alosetron A new drug for pain in diarrhoea-predominant IBS. It is a selective serotonin 5-HT_3 receptor antagonist.

amitriptyline The original tricyclic antidepressant. It is used in low doses for pain in IBS.

anaemia A condition in which the number of red cells circulating in the blood is less than normal.

analgesics Drugs used to reduce pain. 'Simple' analgesics usually refers to medicines that can be bought without a prescription, such as paracetamol, aspirin, ibuprofen and low-dose codeine combined with paracetamol.

anismus An in-co-ordination of the muscles of the pelvis causing difficulty in passing stools. During defecation, the anal sphincter muscles have to relax to allow the stool to pass. In anismus, they may actually tighten, acting against the other pelvic floor muscles and the rectum, which are trying to push the stool out. Also called pelvic floor dyssynergia.

anterior cingulate cortex The part of the brain that is involved with the emotional response to sensations.

antibodies Protein-based molecules made by the immune system to bind on to foreign molecules. Different types of antibody exist to bring about different types of immune reaction.

anticholinergic Relates to drugs that oppose the actions of the parasympathetic nervous system.

antispasmodics Medications, mostly plant extracts, that reduce bowel spasm.

ascites Fluid accumulating in the abdominal cavity.

autonomic nervous system The part of the nervous system of the higher life forms that is not consciously controlled. It is commonly divided into two subsystems that usually act in opposite ways: the sympathetic and parasympathetic nervous systems.

barium A white substance that shows up on X-rays and can be swallowed to outline the stomach (barium meal) or introduced via the anus to outline the colon (barium enema).

benign Relating to a tumour, it means that it will not invade adjacent tissues and will not deposit itself in other parts of the body.

caecum The part of the large bowel into which the small bowel empties. It is positioned in the lower right quadrant of the abdomen.

Candida A yeast. It commonly lives in the large bowel and mouth. It occasionally overgrows, causing thrush.

chronic This usually means of slow onset and lasting a long time.

coeliac disease A disease caused by an immune reaction to gluten, a constituent of wheat.

cognitive behavioural therapy A treatment in which people are taught to identify negative thoughts and behaviours and substitute them with positive ones.

colic When used to describe a pain, it implies severe spasms occurring at regular intervals with some relief between the spasms.

colitis Inflammation of the colon (large bowel).

colonoscopy Examination of the colon using an endoscope.

Crohn's disease An inflammatory condition of unknown cause affecting any part of the gut.

diverticular disease A common finding after middle age. Small pouches bulge outwards from the wall of the colon.

dysmotility Abnormal movement. It usually refers to unco-ordinated muscular activity in a hollow organ such as the stomach.

dyspepsia Indigestion symptoms related to the oesophagus, stomach or duodenum, for example such as heartburn and upper abdominal pain.

dyssynergia of pelvic floor See *anismus*.

endoscopy A general term describing the examination of a hollow organ using a flexible telescopic tube. It is sometimes used to mean the same as gastroscopy.

epidemiology The study of how often medical conditions occur in different groups of people.

epigastrium The region of the abdomen in the midline above the umbilicus.

flexible sigmoidoscopy Endoscopic examination of the lower 50 centimetres of the large bowel.

functional This means that the condition arises from normal function and does not signify any damage.

gastrocolic reflex The reflex increase in bowel activity that occurs when the stomach is distended with food.

gastro-oesophageal reflux disease Reflux of acid back from the stomach into the oesophagus. It usually manifests as heartburn. Sometimes it is just referred to as 'reflux'. It may be denoted as GORD in the UK, or GERD in the USA.

gastroscopy Endoscopic examination of the upper gastrointestinal tract: the oesophagus, stomach and duodenum.

Giardia A one-cell organism that infects the small bowel, causing persistent diarrhoea.

Helicobacter pylori A one-cell organism that infects the stomach, predisposing to ulcers and cancer.

IBS-A IBS with a stool pattern alternating between diarrhoea and constipation. Also denoted by IBS-M (mixed).

IBS-C IBS with a stool pattern dominated by constipation.

IBS-D IBS with a stool pattern dominated by diarrhoea.

IBS-PI IBS occurring post (following) a gastrointestinal infection.

IBS-U Unsubtyped IBS, denoting the condition in people with IBS symptoms but an insufficient change in the character of their stools to fit into any of the other categories.

ileocaecal valve The structure at the opening of the small bowel into the large bowel. It is designed to limit backflow of the contents.

impaction Almost total blockage of the bowel with stool.

inflammation A complex process involving a reaction to infection or damage. It is characterised by an increased blood supply causing redness, a leakage of fluid from the blood vessels causing swelling, and the presence of cells from the immune system to destroy or remove harmful material.

inflammatory bowel disease The general term for disease of the gut characterised by inflammation of unknown cause. It includes ulcerative colitis and Crohn's disease.

insula A part of the brain thought to be involved in assessing the intensity of pain.

lactase An enzyme in the small bowel designed to break down lactose.

lactose The sugar of dairy products.

left iliac fossa The lower left quadrant of the abdomen.

loperamide A drug used to slow propulsion through the intestine.

malabsorption Failure to absorb.

malignant When applied to tumours, it means that they invade adjacent structures and can deposit in other parts of the body.

melaena Tarry black, loose and shiny stools caused by bleeding from high in the gastrointestinal tract.

motility Gastrointestinal motility is defined by the movements of the digestive system, and the transit of the contents within it.

mucosa The lining of the bowel.

mucus A slime produced in the gut that lubricates and protects the mucosa. The passage of mucus with the stool is normal in some people and common in IBS.

NSAIDs Non-steroidal anti-inflammatory drugs, such as aspirin, ibuprofen and diclofenac.

oestrogen The main female hormone.

overflow diarrhoea Diarrhoea that occurs when the bowel is actually full of stool. Large lumps of hard stool fill the bowel and do not pass along it. Soft stool and water then pass around and between the lumps to give the effect of diarrhoea. The bowel literally overflows.

parasympathetic One of two divisions of the autonomic nervous system. It conserves energy as it slows the heart rate, increases intestinal and glandular activity, and relaxes sphincter muscles in the gastrointestinal tract. It uses only acetylcholine as its neurotransmitter, and it can be blocked by drugs with anticholinergic activity.

peristalsis Continuous co-ordinated contractions of the muscles of the gut to propel the contents along.

pharmacology The scientific study of medicinal drugs. It explains how drugs work and their effects on body systems.

physiology The scientific study of bodily functions; how the various systems of the body work together to maintain normal function.

placebo An inert substance given as a medicine for its suggestive effect.

polyps Small, mushroom-like growths on the bowel wall that are usually benign.

probiotics Preparations of living organisms that are thought to be beneficial to health.

progesterone A female hormone that, with oestrogen, prepares the uterus to receive a fertilised egg.

pubo-rectalis A pelvic muscle that forms a sling around the rectum.

right iliac fossa The right lower quadrant of the abdomen.

senna A popular herbal stimulant laxative.

serotonin A chemical used to relay information between some nerve cells and adjacent cells (neurotransmitter) found extensively in the gastro-intestinal tract and in the brain. Also called 5-hydroxytryptamine (5-HT).

somatosensory cortex The part of the brain concerned with the spatial localisation of sensations.

SSRIs Selective serotonin reuptake inhibitors, a group of antidepressants that increase serotonin levels and so amplify the effects of nerve cells that use serotonin.

steatorrhoea Diarrhoea with a high fat content. Yellowish in colour, it smells offensive, floats and is difficult to flush away.

sympathetic A part of the nervous system that is concerned with regulating the function of internal organs, particularly during times of emotional or physical stress ('fight or flight' response). Adrenaline levels rise, and the blood supply is diverted away from the gut and kidneys and towards the muscles.

syndrome A syndrome is a collection of symptoms and signs that tend to occur and run together, producing a recognisable ailment. It may have a variety of causes or no definable cause.

tegaserod A new drug for pain in constipation-predominant IBS. A selective serotonin type 4 (5-HT$_4$) receptor partial agonist.

terminal ileum The last part of the small bowel. It enters the caecum in the lower right quadrant of the abdomen.

tricyclic antidepressants A class of antidepressant drug first used in the 1950s. Although constipating in normal doses, they can be very useful for the pain of IBS when used in low doses.

ulcerative colitis An inflammatory condition of unknown cause affecting only the large bowel.

urgency of stool Sometimes just called urgency. The need to really rush to the toilet.

visceral Pertaining to the internal organs, such as the gastrointestinal system.

visceral hypersensitivity The concept of enhanced perception, or enhanced responsiveness within the gut – even to normal events.

Appendix 1 – Useful resources

GENERAL ORGANISATIONS AND WEBSITES WITH INFORMATION ON IBS AND RELATED TOPICS

Go Ask Alice!
Website: www.goaskalice.columbia.edu
A question and answer Internet service produced by Alice!, Columbia University's Health Promotion Program — a division of Health Services at Columbia. 'Alice!' answers questions about relationships, sexuality, sexual health, emotional health, fitness, nutrition, alcohol, nicotine and other drugs, and general health.

HealingWell
Website: www.healingwell.com
A large site concentrating on natural remedies for chronic conditions including IBS.

Medicine Net
Website: www.medicinenet.com
An American general medical site.

Patient.co.uk
Website: www.patient.co.uk
A searchable UK medical site, with information on most medical conditions and multiple links.

Prodigy
Sowerby Centre for Health Informatics at Newcastle
(SCHIN Ltd)
Bede House
All Saints Business Centre
Newcastle upon Tyne NE1 2ES
Tel: 0191 243 6100
E-mail: prodigy-enquiries@schin.co.uk
Website: www.prodigy.nhs.uk
Useful leaflets on a wide range of conditions.

UpToDate
Website: http://patients.uptodate.com
The patient information part of this website is free and contains authoritative detailed articles on most medical conditions.

Wikipedia
Website: http://en.wikipedia.org
A free on-line general encyclopaedia.

Wrong diagnosis

Website: www.wrongdiagnosis.com
An interesting site that allows you to search for information on specific diseases or symptoms. There is an emphasis on misdiagnosis and how errors occur, with lists of alternative diagnoses. Although a lot of information is provided, it will understandably be not quite enough for a lay person to distinguish one condition from another.

GASTROENTEROLOGY ORGANISATIONS AND SITES

American Gastroenterological Association

Email: member@gastro.org
Website: www.gastro.org
The 'Patient Center' link has numerous articles on most aspects of gastroenterological and liver diseases.

Celiac Sprue Association of the United States of America

Website: www.csaceliacs.org
The Celiac Sprue Association is a member-based, non-profit support organisation dedicated to helping individuals with coeliac disease and dermatitis herpetiformis and their families worldwide through information, education and research.

Celiac Disease Foundation

Website: www.celiac.org
The Celiac Disease Foundation provides support, information and assistance to people affected by coeliac disease and dermatitis herpetiformis. It increases awareness among the general public and works closely with healthcare professionals and the pharmaceutical and medical industries.

Coeliac UK

Suites A–D
Octagon Court
High Wycombe
Buckinghamshire HP11 2HS
Tel: 01949 437 278
Helpline: 0870 444 8804
Website: www.coeliac.co.uk
Coeliac UK aims to improve the lives of people living with the condition through support, campaigning and research so that the needs of people with coeliac disease and dermatitis herpetiformis are universally recognised and met. The society also provides a free dietetic and food helpline for people struggling with diagnosis and management of their condition. In addition, they can provide helpful leaflets and books, and run voluntary groups around the UK.

IBSPage.com – The IBS Page

Website: www.ibspage.com
A large list of websites on irritable bowel syndrome.

US Department of Agriculture, Nutrient Data Laboratory

Website: www.ars.usda.gov/ba/bhnrc/ndl, www.ars.usda.gov/nutrientdata

A searchable and downloadable free database of the nutrient data for a huge list of foods.

Yorktest Laboratories Ltd

G3
York Science Park
York YO19 5DQ
Tel: 01904 410410
Website: www.yorktest.com

A commercial site that sends out blood-based allergy testing kits. Blood from a finger prick is returned to the laboratory, which provides a report.

CORE

3 St Andrews Place
London
NW1 4LB
Tel: 020 7486 0341
Email: info@corecharity.org.uk
Website: www.corecharity.org.uk

CORE is the working name of the Digestive Disorders Foundation. The website provides patient information leaflets on a variety of gastrointestinal disorders, and a glossary of medical terms related to gastroenterology.

IBS-SPECIFIC SITES

International Foundation for Functional Gastrointestinal Disorders

Email: iffgd@iffgd.org
Website: www.iffgd.org/index.html

The IFFGD, founded in 1991, is a registered non-profit-making educational and research organisation. It addresses the issues surrounding life with gastrointestinal functional and motility disorders and increases awareness about these disorders among the general public, researchers, regulators and the clinical care community. It has a large and authoritative website with numerous detailed articles on IBS and other functional diseases.

IBS Group

Email: ibs@ibsgroup.org
Website: www.ibsgroup.org

This is an American self-help and support group site. It gives access to up-to-date information, including videos, as well as chat groups and weblinks.

IBS Network
Unit 5
53 Mowbray Street
Sheffield
South Yorkshire S3 8EN
*(All written enquiries must be
accompanied by an SAE)*
Tel: 0114 272 3253
Helpline: 0114 272 3253
*(Mon–Fri 6–8 pm, Sat 10–12 am;
calls answered by IBS specialist
nurses)*
Email: info@ibsnetwork.org.uk
Website: www.ibsnetwork.org.uk
*The IBS Network is a UK national
charity offering advice, information
and support. It has a large informative
website now including the IBS
Network Self Management
Programme. This consists of 11
modules, adaptable for individual
study on your computer, dealing with
every aspect of IBS. These are very
readable and full of useful suggestions
and links.*

IBS Research Update
Website: www.ibs-research-update.org.uk
*This is the website of the IBS
Research Appeal, a charitable research
programme run by medical
practitioners who treat sufferers of
IBS on a daily basis at their clinic at
the Central Middlesex Hospital,
London NW10.*

Rome Criteria
Website: www.romecriteria.org
*This is the official website of the Rome
criteria for IBS. It contains links to
the 2006 issue of the journal
Gastroenterology summarising the
research from which the criteria and
definitions of IBS were devised.*

IBS Tales
Website: www.ibstales.com
*Read the personal stories of IBS
sufferers and share your own
experiences. A fascinating and moving
site for anyone with IBS, their
relatives and doctors.*

Bowel Control
Website: www.bowelcontrol.org.uk
*A site based at St Mark's Hospital,
London, giving clear and concise
explanations and advice for people
with faecal incontinence.*

**Irritable Bowel Syndrome
Treatment**
Website: www.irritable-bowel-syndrome
Easily accessible tips and suggestions.

PSYCHOLOGICAL SERVICES

British Psychological Society
St Andrews House
48 Princess Road East
Leicester
East Midlands LE1 7DR
Tel: 0116 254 9568
Email: enquiry@bps.org.uk
Website: www.bps.org.uk/home-page.cfm
This gives information on properly qualified clinical psychologists who practise cognitive behavioural therapy.

London Clinic of Psychoanalysis
Byron House
112A Shirland Road
London. W9 2EQ
Tel: 020 7563 5002
Email: clinic@iopa.org.uk
Website:
www.psychoanalysis.org.uk/clinic.htm
For psychoanalytic therapy.

COMPLEMENTARY THERAPY

British Medical Acupuncture Society
BMAS House
3 Winnington Court
Northwich
Cheshire CW8 1AQ
Tel: 01606 786782
Email: Admin@medical-acupuncture.org.uk
Website: www.medical-acupuncture.co.uk
The BMAS was formed in 1980 as an association of medical practitioners interested in acupuncture. There are now over 2300 members who use acupuncture in hospital or general practice. The society promotes the use of acupuncture as a therapy following orthodox medical diagnosis by suitably trained practitioners. It encourages the use and scientific understanding of acupuncture within medicine and seeks to enhance the education and training of suitably qualified practitioners, and to promote high standards of working practice in acupuncture.

**British Society
of Clinical Hypnosis**
125 Queensgate
Bridlington
East Yorkshire YO16 7JQ
Tel: 01262 403103
Email: sec@bsch.org.uk
Website: www.bsch.org.uk
*A body whose aim is to promote
and assure high standards in the
profession of hypnotherapy. From
the website, you can search for a
hypnotist in your area, learn about
the code of conduct expected from
members of the society and learn
more about hypnotherapy in practice.*

**National Register
of Hypnotherapists
and Psychotherapists**
Suite B
12 Cross Street
Nelson
Lancashire BB9 7EN
Tel: 01282 716839
Email: nrhp@btconnect.com
Website: www.nrhp.co.uk
*The NRHP is a leading, non-profit-
making register of qualified hypno-
psychotherapists. The site contains
information to help you decide
whether you need the services of
one of the society's members. It also
holds a database of hypnotherapists
throughout the country and provides
a free referral service for those seeking
a reputable practitioner.*

**The Prince's Foundation
for Integrated Health**
33–41 Dallington Street
London
EC1V 0BB
Tel: 020 3119 3100
Fax: 020 3119 3101
Email: info@fih.org.uk
*The Prince's Foundation for Integrated
Health is dedicated to helping people,
practitioners and communities to
create an integrated approach to
health and well-being. The site
includes a 55-page guide for patients
seeking complementary health care.*

**The UK Register
of IBS Therapists**
Website: www.ibs-register.co.uk
*A listing of UK hypnotherapists
specialising in treating IBS with
hypnotherapy.*

SELECTED BOOKS

IBS: A Complete Guide to Relief from Irritable Bowel Syndrome, by Christine P. Dancey and Susan Backhouse, published by Constable & Robinson, London (2003).

The Sufferers' Guide to Coping with IBS, published by the IBS Appeal with medical notes by Dr DBA Silk, available from www.ibs-research-update.org.uk *Practical advice on living with irritable bowel syndrome, including foods that help and hinder in the experience of sufferers.*

IBS: Take Control, by Christine P. Dancey, Claire L. Rutter, Bernard Atherton and Steve Chadburn, published by Constable and Robinson, London (1997).
A book that approaches IBS from a psychological viewpoint aiming to increase people's insight into their condition and enhance their coping skills.

Fast Facts: Irritable Bowel Syndrome by Kenneth W. Heaton and W. Grant Thompson, published by Health Press, Oxford (2003).
Although aimed at doctors, this small paperback gives a well-written account of the key facts and concepts of IBS.

Appendix 2 – Medicines available 'over the counter' for treating IBS in the UK

Laxatives

Generic name	Common brand names (available without prescription)	Onset of action	Comments
Bulk-forming laxatives			Fibre preparations available over the counter
Ispaghula husk (psyllium)	Regulan, Fybogel, Metamucil (USA)	12–72 hours, but be prepared to give it longer	This is usually available as granules. It increases bloating, at least initially. Drink plenty of water
Sterculia	Normacol, Normacol Plus	12–72 hours	This is a gum obtained from *Sterculia* plants
Methylcellulose	Celevac, Citrucel (USA)	12–72 hours	This is a synthetic soluble fibre, designed to produce less bacterial breakdown so less wind. It is available as tablets or a liquid
Osmotic laxatives			Hold water within the bowel

Laxatives *continued*

Generic name	Common brand names (available without prescription)	Onset of action	Comments
Lactulose	Duphalac, Lactugal, Regulose	Usually 0.5–3 hours, but can take as long as 24–48 hours	This comes as a sweet-tasting syrup. It can be diluted with water, fruit juice or milk, or taken in a food. It often causes bloating and wind. Lactulose is a relatively weak laxative
Magnesium hydroxide	Milk of Magnesia, Cream of Magnesia	0.5–3 hours	This is available as a liquid suspension. It can be potent and rapidly acting. Take plenty of fluids. It is to be avoided in renal failure
Magnesium sulphate	Epsom Salts, Andrews Liver Salts or Original	0.4–3 hours	This is more potent than magnesium hydroxide. It can cause severe bloating and sudden diarrhoea. Andrews Salts also contain sodium bicarbonate and citric acid so work as an antacid too
Polyethylene glycols	Movicol, Idrolax	1–2 hours but can be much longer in some people	This comes as a sachet of powder that is taken with water. It is probably as effective and more palatable than magnesium hydroxide

Laxatives *continued*

Generic name	Common brand names (available without prescription)	Onset of action	Comments
Emollient laxatives			Soften the stool
Liquid paraffin	Liquid paraffin oral emulsion	6–8 hours	This softens the stool and lubricates the intestine, but anal leakage of paraffin acts as an irritant
Docusate sodium	Dioctyl, Docusol, Norglass Micro-enema	12–72 hours when taken orally. A few minutes to 15 minutes as an enema	This has some bowel-stimulating activity as well as softening the stool. It is relatively mild
Stimulant laxatives			Stimulate muscular contraction in the bowel, which can be painful
Senna	Senokot, Manevac, Ex-lax Senna	8–12 hours	This is available as tablets, granules or a syrup
Bisacodyl	Dulco-lax (bisacodyl)	6–10 hours when taken orally; 15–30 minutes as a suppository	This comes as tablets or suppositories. It is probably more reliable than senna
Sodium picosulphate	Dulco-lax (sodium picosulphate), Laxoberal	6–10 hours	This is a potent stimulant laxative available as an elixir or tablets

Enemas and suppositories

Enemas and suppositories are particularly useful for clearing the rectum.
They are the best laxatives to use when the rectum is full of hard stool.
They usually work within a few minutes to half an hour.

Generic name	Common brand names (available without prescription)	Comments
Glycerol suppositories	Glycerin suppositories	Draws water into the rectum from the blood supply, stimulating defecation
Bisacodyl suppositories	Dulco-lax (bisacodyl 10 mg suppository), Dulco-lax suppository for children 5 mg	Stimulates the muscles of the rectum
Phosphate suppository	Carbalax	Stimulates a bowel movement by distending the rectum. The phosphate works by drawing water into the rectum from the blood supply. The suppository also contains sodium bicarbonate, which reacts with the water to produce carbon dioxide gas, further distending the rectum and causing the muscles to contract
Phosphate enemas	Fleet Enema, Fletchers' Enema	
Sodium citrate	Micralax and Relaxit Micro-enema	Work in the same way as the phosphate enemas, but with a much smaller volume. Are therefore easier to use
Arachis oil	Fletchers' Arachis Oil Retention Enema	This softens hard stool in the lower bowel. It comes only as an enema. Do not use it if you are allergic to nuts

Opiate-based medications used to treat diarrhoea

Generic name	Brand names	Comment
Loperamide	Arrett capsules, Boots Diareze, Diasorb, Diocalm Ultra, Imodium (including Imodium liquid), Imodium Plus, Normaloe	This is an opiate-based drug that acts selectively on the gut. As a result, it has little or no analgesic effect. There is also little or no risk of dependence. Drowsiness may be a side effect in large doses, but most people are virtually unaffected. A single dose of loperamide can remain effective for 24 hours
Diphenoxylate and atropine	Lomotil	Diphenoxylate is similar to loperamide. The small dose of atropine in the mixture also slows the bowel by blocking the activity of another set of nerves (cholinergic nerves) that would otherwise increase bowel activity. In larger doses, atropine will cause unpleasant side effects such as a dry mouth and blurred vision. This means that Lomotil cannot be taken in large doses
Codeine and dihydrocodeine	These are available over the counter in small doses, usually combined with paracetamol	These are opiate-based medications used mainly as analgesics. They slow the bowel effectively but are likely to cause drowsiness. Tolerance is a problem, which means they may become less effective over time. It is possible to become addicted to codeine

Adsorbents to treat diarrhoea

Generic name	Brand names	Comment
Kaolin	Kaolin mixture, kaoline and morphine	A traditional remedy for diarrhoea. The kaolin absorbs some of the water in the bowel. Not as effective as loperamide. It can be combined with a small dose of morphine, an opiate that slows the bowel, but this gives a risk of drowsiness
Attapulgite	Diocalm Dual Action (with morphine)	Attapulgite is a clay. It is said to absorb excess water and possibly bacteria. It is being discontinued in the USA because of fear that it may contain lead. It is still available in the UK combined with a small dose of morphine
Charcoal	Medicinal or activated charcoal	Charcoal has a high surface area to volume ratio and absorbs many gases and to some extent liquids

Other over-the-counter medications used in diarrhoea

Generic name	Brand names	Comment
Bismuth subsalicylate	Pepto-Bismol	Effective for mild diarrhoea, but large doses may be necessary
Rehydration salts	Dioralyte	These do not significantly reduce the quantity of diarrhoea. They are used to prevent the dehydration caused by severe diarrhoea

Antispasmodics

Generic name	Brand names	Comment
Peppermint oil	Colpermin, Mintec	Relax the muscle of the bowel. May also help with flatulence. May cause heartburn
Alverine citrate	Spasmonal	Relaxes the muscle of the bowel
Mebeverine	Colofac IBS, Fybogel Mebeverine	One of the most commonly prescribed antispasmodics for IBS
Hyoscine	Buscopan IBS	Anticholinergic, so may cause constipation or blurred vision and dry mouth
Dicycloverine (previously called dicyclomine)	Merbentyl, Kolanticon gel (this also contains antacids, which neutralise acid in the stomach)	Anticholinergic, so may cause constipation or blurred vision and dry mouth

Other useful medications available over the counter

Generic name	Brand names	Comment
Domperidone	Motilium	Good for nausea. Safe and free from side effects
Omeprazole	Zanprol	Reduces acid production by the stomach. Very effective but can take several hours to work
Ranitidine Famotidine	Zantac Pepcid AC	Reduce acid production by the stomach. Not as effective as omeprazole but work more quickly

Index

Have you found *Irritable Bowel Syndrome: Answers at your fingertips* useful and practical? If so, you may be interested in other books from Class Publishing.

Heart Health:
Answers at your fingertips   £17.99

Dr Graham Jackson

This practical handbook, written by a leading cardiologist, answers all your questions about heart conditions. It tells you all about you and your heart; how to keep your heart healthy, or – if it has been affected by heart disease – how to make it as strong as possible.

> *'Those readers who want to know more about the various treatments for heart disease will be much enlightened.'*
> DR JAMES LE FANU, *The Daily Telegraph*

Beating Depression   £17.99

Dr Stefan Cembrowicz and Dr Dorcas Kingham

Depression is one of most common illnesses in the world – affecting up to one in four people at some time in their lives. *Beating Depression* shows sufferers and their families that they are not alone, and offers tried and tested techniques for overcoming depression.

> *'A sympathetic and understanding guide.'*
> MARJORIE WALLACE, Chief Executive, SANE

Type 1 Diabetes:
Answers at your fingertips   £14.99

Type 2 Diabetes:
Answers at your fingertips   £14.99

Both by Dr Charles Fox and Dr Anne Kilvert

The latest edition of our bestselling reference guide for people with diabetes has now been split into two books covering the two distinct forms of the disease. These books maintain the popular question-and-answer format, to provide practical advice on every aspect of living with the condition, and give you the knowledge and reassurance you need to deal confidently with your diabetes.

Food Allergies: Enjoying Life
with a Severe Food Allergy   £19.99

Tanya Wright with Medical Adviser, Dr Joanne Clough

Expert dietitian Tanya Wright combines her professional and personal experience of severe food allergy to give you a unique source of practical advice. In this indispensable handbook you will learn what it is safe for you to eat and what you must avoid. This book shows you how to carry on enjoying life and food, despite your allergy.

> *'Required reading for those with food allergies.'*
> DAVID READING, Director,
> The Anaphylaxis Campaign

The Back Pain Book   £17.99

Mike Hage

Nearly two thirds of adults in the UK have had experience of back pain. Now there's hope – and help – for the sufferer. This book offers guidance on how to use posture and movement to ease, relieve and prevent back pain.

> *'The book is the most comprehensive book I have come across as a self-help guide to back problems.'*
> RICHARD PERRY, London

Migraine:
Answers at your fingertips   £14.99

Dr Manuela Fontebasso

Written by an experienced GP with a special interest in headache and migraine, this book acknowledges the uniqueness of every sufferer's experience. Communication between patient and professional is crucial if this complex condition is to be addressed and the best treatment prescribed.

This book will help you understand the nature of your headache, and give you the confidence to be involved in all areas of decision making.

PRIORITY ORDER FORM

Cut out or photocopy this form and send it (post free in the UK) to:

Class Publishing   **Tel: 01256 302 699**
FREEPOST 16705   **Fax: 01256 812 558**
Macmillan Distribution
Basingstoke RG21 6ZZ

Please send me urgently   *Post included*
(tick below)   *price per copy (UK only)*

☐ **Irritable Bowel Syndrome: Answers at your fingertips**   £20.99
   (ISBN 978 1 85959 156 7)

☐ **Heart Health: Answers at your fingertips** (ISBN 978 1885959 157 4)   £20.99

☐ **Beating Depression** (ISBN 978 1 85959 150 5)   £20.99

☐ **Type 1 Diabetes: Answers at your fingertips** (ISBN 9781 85959 175 8)   £17.99

☐ **Type 2 Diabetes: Answers at your fingertips** (ISBN 9781 85959 176 5)   £17.99

☐ **Food Allergies** (ISBN 978 1 85959 146 8)   £22.99

☐ **The Back Pain Book** (ISBN 978 1 85959 124 6)   £20.99

☐ **Migraine: Answers at your fingertips** (ISBN 978 1 85959 149 9)   £17.99

                                                   TOTAL _____

Easy ways to pay

Cheque: I enclose a cheque payable to Class Publishing for £ _____

Credit card: Please debit my ☐ Mastercard   ☐ Visa   ☐ Amex

Number _____ Expiry date _____

Name _____

My address for delivery is _____

_____

Town _____ County _____ Postcode _____

Telephone number (*in case of query*) _____

Credit card billing address if different from above _____

_____

Town _____ County _____ Postcode _____

Class Publishing's guarantee: remember that if, for any reason, you are not satisfied with these books, we will refund all your money, without any questions asked. Prices and VAT rates may be altered for reasons beyond our control.